D0819417

Nursing Research
and **Evidence-Based**
Practice

Ten Steps to Success

Rebecca Keele, PhD, APHN-BC
Associate Professor, Nursing
School of Nursing
New Mexico State University
Las Cruces, New Mexico

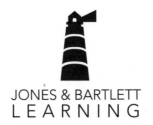

JONES & BARTLETT
LEARNING

World Headquarters

Jones & Bartlett Learning
40 Tall Pine Drive
Sudbury, MA 01776
978-443-5000
info@jblearning.com
www.jblearning.com

Jones & Bartlett Learning
Canada
6339 Ormindale Way
Mississauga, Ontario L5V 1J2
Canada

Jones & Bartlett Learning
International
Barb House, Barb Mews
London W6 7PA
United Kingdom

Jones & Bartlett Learning books and products are available through most bookstores and online booksellers. To contact Jones & Bartlett Learning directly, call 800-832-0034, fax 978-443-8000, or visit our website, www.jblearning.com.

Substantial discounts on bulk quantities of Jones & Bartlett Learning publications are available to corporations, professional associations, and other qualified organizations. For details and specific discount information, contact the special sales department at Jones & Bartlett Learning via the above contact information or send an email to specialsales@jblearning.com.

Copyright © 2011 by Jones & Bartlett Learning, LLC

All rights reserved. No part of the material protected by this copyright may be reproduced or utilrights reserved. No part of the material protected by this copyright may be reproduced or utilized in any form, electronic or mechanical, including photocopying, recording, or by any information storage and retrieval system, without written permission from the copyright owner.

The author, editor, and publisher have made every effort to provide accurate information. However, they are not responsible for errors, omissions, or for any outcomes related to the use of the contents of this book and take no responsibility for the use of the products and procedures described. Treatments and side-effects described in this book may not be applicable to all people; likewise, some people may require a dose or experience a side-effect that is not described herein. Drugs and medical devices are discussed that may have limited availability controlled by the Food and Drug Administration (FDA) for use only in a research study or clinical trial. Research, clinical practice, and government regulations often change the accepted standard in this field. When consideration is being given to use of any drug in the clinical setting, the health care provider or reader is responsible for determining FDA status of the drug, reading the package insert, and reviewing prescribing information for the most up-to-date recommendations on dose, precautions, and contraindications, and determining the appropriate usage for the product. This is especially important in the case of drugs that are new or seldom used.

Production Credits

Publisher: Kevin Sullivan
Acquisitions Editor: Amy Sibley
Associate Editor: Patricia Donnelly
Editorial Assistant: Rachel Shuster
Production Assistant: Sara Fowles
Associate Marketing Manager:
  Katie Hennessy
V.P., Manufacturing and Inventory Control:
  Therese Connell
Composition: DataStream Content
  Solutions, LLC
Cover Image: © Kheng Guan Toh/ShutterStock, Inc.
Printing and Binding: Malloy, Inc.
Cover Printing: Malloy, Inc.

Library of Congress Cataloging-in-Publication Data
Keele, Rebecca.
    Nursing research and evidence-based practice : ten steps to success / Rebecca Keele.
      p. ; cm.
    Includes bibliographical references and index.
    ISBN 978-0-7637-8058-6 (pbk.)
    1. Nursing--Research.   2. Evidence-based nursing.   I. Title.
    [DNLM: 1. Nursing Research—methods.   2. Evidence-Based Nursing.   3. Research Design.
WY 20.5 K26n 2011]
    RT81.5.K44 2011
    610.73072—dc22
                                                                            2010018671

6048

Printed in the United States of America
14 13 12 11   10 9 8 7 6 5 4 3 2

Dedication

This book is dedicated to my children, Kristan, Michael, Joshua, Haley, and Andrew, who make my life meaningful and fun.

Contents

Preface . . . . *ix*

Acknowledgments . . . . *xi*

CHAPTER 1   Beginning Tips on Surviving Nursing Research and
Evidence-Based Nursing Practice *1*

What Is Nursing Research? 1

What Is Research Utilization? 4

What Is Evidence-Based Nursing Practice? 5

Comparing Research and Evidence-Based Practice 6

Debunking the Myths 7

Overcoming the Barriers 10

The Big "So What?" 14

References 15

CHAPTER 2   The Quantitative Research Process *17*

Problem Statement 17

Literature Review 18

Theoretical/Conceptual Framework 19

Research Questions/Hypotheses 21

Confounding/Extraneous Variables 23

Research Design 24

Sampling 24

Data Collection 27

Data Analysis 30

Findings/Recommendations 31

Strengths and Limitations 31

Dissemination of Findings 32

The Big "So What?" 32

References 33

CHAPTER 3 Quantitative Versus Qualitative Research, or Both? *35*

Nursing Research Worldviews 35

Quantitative Designs 37

Qualitative Designs 44

Mixed Methods 50

Quantitative Versus Qualitative Versus Both
(Mixed Methods)? 51

The Big "So What?" 51

References 52

CHAPTER 4 Data Analysis *53*

Descriptive Statistics 55

Inferential Statistics 62

Choosing the Appropriate Statistical Test 66

Interpreting Statistical Tests 71

The Big "So What?" 72

References 73

CHAPTER 5 Implementing Evidence-Based Nursing Practice:
An Overview *75*

Getting Started 75

Identification of the Clinical Practice Problem 83

Collecting and Appraising the Evidence 83

Reading and Critically Analyzing Empirical Research 85

Summarizing Across the Evidence 85

Integrating the Evidence with Clinical Expertise and
Client Preferences and Values 86

Developing the Proposed Practice Change in Detail. 86

Feasibility Issues 88

Evaluating the Practice Change 90

Marketing the Practice Change 91

Strategies for Successful Implementation 91

Sustainability of Practice Change 91

The Big "So What?" 92

References. 92

CHAPTER 6   Reading and Critically Analyzing Empirical
Research Studies *95*

Ten Easy (Or Will Become Easy) Steps to Analyzing
Quantitative Empirical Research. 95

Quantitative Sample Article 1. 98

Quantitative Sample Article 2. 101

Ten Steps in Analyzing Qualitative Research Studies 104

Qualitative Sample Article 1 104

Qualitative Sample Article 2 109

The Big "So What?" 112

References. 112

Appendix 6A 113

Appendix 6B 123

Appendix 6C 141

Appendix 6D 171

CHAPTER 7   Now It Is Your Turn to Analyze Research. *187*

Qualitative Research Study Example Using the
Ten Steps. 187

Quantitative Research Study Example Using the
Ten Steps. 193

Qualitative Study Example for You to Do on Your Own . . 198

Quantitative Study Example for You to Do on Your Own. . 201

The Big "So What?" 205

References. 205

CHAPTER 8   Ethics in Research and Evidence-Based
                Nursing Practice. *207*

                Ethics in Nursing Research. 207
                Ethics in Evidence-Based Nursing Practice 222
                References. 226

CHAPTER 9   Evidence-Based Nursing Practice Projects:
                Putting It All Together. *229*

                Time to Get Doing 229
                References. 248

CHAPTER 10 Planned Change in Evidence-Based Nursing Practice *251*

                Rogers' Diffusion of Innovations Theory 252
                Rogers' Diffusion of Innovations Applied to
                Evidence-Based Nursing Practice 256
                References. 262

                Index *265*

Preface

This evidence-based nursing practice textbook is based on the idea that evidence-based nursing practice (EBNP) is not an option for practicing nurses but a requirement to ensure quality patient care. Based on this premise, the goal of writing this textbook was to make research and evidence-based nursing practice less painful and hopefully more interesting. As a result, it is hoped that practicing nurses and/or nursing students will develop a positive perception of research and evidence-based practice and be more motivated in using it with their clients.

To provide consistency and simplicity, the textbook incorporates the idea of 10 steps in 10 chapters. A 10-step process is presented for doing EBNP and for analyzing nursing research studies. Evidence-based nursing practice is a popular term used in practice and the academic setting. However, there is a lack of consensus on what it actually means when the concept is applied to practice. This book discusses these issues, along with a presentation of some of the common models used for EBNP. After a discussion on the strengths and limitations of each model, an attempt is made to cut through the confusion and the complexity by suggesting 10 practical steps for doing evidence-based nursing practice.

The goal of this textbook is not to make the reader a nurse scientist, but to provide the tools to critically appraise all types of evidence and integrate this evidence with patient preferences and values and expert opinion. Focus is on knowledge of the research process, quantitative versus qualitative research designs, ethical issues, basic knowledge of some of the most common empirical analyses, appraisal of evidence, and integration of the evidence into nursing practice.

This book differs in its approach and content from traditional nursing research textbooks. While including all of the core ingredients of a traditional nursing research textbook, it emphasizes a practical how-to approach in doing EBNP. Several full examples of nursing research article critiques and evidence-based nursing practice projects are included. The textbook is organized to lead the skeptic or insecure reader in a way that reduces the negative perceptions of research and evidence-based nursing practice.

Chapter 1 addresses many of the myths and negative perceptions about EBNP and argues for the absolute necessity of incorporating evidence-based nursing practice into one's own practice. This chapter also provides an introduction into the research process and the evidence-based nursing practice process. Chapter 2 provides more detail about the quantitative research process, and Chapter 3 addresses qualitative research, how to decide on methodologies and research designs, and the option of possibly using both. Chapter 4 is a very basic presentation of the most common statistical analyses seen in nursing research studies, as well as strategies for selecting appropriate statistical analyses. Chapter 5 is an overview of evidence-based nursing practice, whereas Chapter 6 is focused on reading and analyzing both quantitative and qualitative research studies using full examples. Chapter 7 again focuses on analyzing research studies but encourages the reader to do more on their own and then compare their findings to the textbook. Chapter 8 covers not only ethics in nursing research but also ethics as it applies to evidence-based nursing practice. The primary goal of Chapter 9 is to pull all of the pieces presented thus far together to develop actual evidence-based nursing practice projects. Lastly, Chapter 10 puts the icing on the cake by addressing the critical issue of how to facilitate behavioral change. Without planned change, the total evidence-based nursing practice project/process will be set up for failure.

Thus, the unique features of this textbook include the following:

- Simple approach to analyzing nursing research and doing evidence-based nursing practice
- Attempt to debunk the myths that many nursing students and practicing nurses have in regard to research and EBNP
- A section on ethical implications of EBNP
- A chapter on planned change and how it relates to EBNP
- Several full examples of research article critiques using the 10-step guidelines provided by the book
- Reduction of content on nursing research from the nice-to-know to the have-to-know core content
- Full examples of evidence-based nursing practice examples using the 10-step approach provided in this textbook
- Most chapters end with a Big "So What?" bulleted section to provide the essentials from that chapter

The author of this book recognizes the struggles that practicing nurses have in integrating evidence-based nursing practice in their daily work lives. Over 22 years of experience teaching in both undergraduate and graduate programs, seeing nursing students struggle with research terminology and concepts, and frankly not understanding its usefulness to their future practices has led to the writing of this book. As the title indicates, the goal of this book is to make evidence-based nursing practice less painful and more significant in the lives of current practicing nurses and future professional nurses. Ultimately, this will lead to improved quality of patient care, which is why we as nurses do what we do each day.

Acknowledgments

I particularly want to say thank you to my son Joshua, who helped me with my two younger children while I diligently worked on this book. I also thank my two youngest children, Haley and Andrew, for putting up with me during this time.

Beginning Tips on Surviving Nursing Research and Evidence-Based Nursing Practice

WHAT IS NURSING RESEARCH?

Nursing research is a systematic process that uses rigorous guidelines to answer questions about nursing practice. It may involve validating and refining existing knowledge or developing new knowledge. The purpose of nursing research is to provide empirical evidence to support nursing practice, which in turn ultimately affects the care we provide to our clients. Nursing research also contributes to the empirical body of knowledge, criteria necessary for professional status.

The systematic process referred to above implies planning and organization, not chaos; however, it is not without flexibility. Typically, the steps of the research process include:

- Identification of a problem
- Reading the related literature
- Identification of the research question(s) or hypothesis(es)
- Selecting a theoretical framework or creating a conceptual framework
- Deciding on what design will answer the research question/hypothesis the best
- Identification of a reasonable sample
- Deciding on data collection issues
- Who, what, where, when, and how
- Taking into consideration feasibility issues—budget, timeline, availability of participants, expertise of the researcher, materials needed
- Analyzing the data
- Determining findings
- Dissemination of the findings

The above steps provide the structure, but the process allows movement back and forth between the steps as needed to allow for refinement and tweaking of the study. For example, the researcher may want to use an experimental design but may find as they move into sampling that there are not enough available participants to have an adequate sample size to test the proposed intervention. This may require the researcher to change their design to something a little less rigorous. Even though all of the above steps are important, the last one is probably the most critical. Why expend the energy and resources if you never share it with anyone? Following is a short description of each step. More detail will follow in further chapters.

Identification of a Problem

This is usually a researcher's first step and can be one of the most difficult steps. The difficulty usually comes because it can be very challenging to refine the problem statement enough so that it is researchable. Usually, the researcher moves from a broad area of interest such as "health promotion" to a more specific problem such as "compliance with physical activity for Mexican-American adults."

Reading the Related Literature

To assess what is known and what is not known about a particular problem, a review of the literature is necessary. Information from the literature review can guide the researcher regarding what types of studies to conduct. The review guides the researcher as to selection of type and level of design, age group, gender, ethnicity, etc., or even if the study should be done at all depending on whether enough knowledge already exists to make a practice change.

Identification of the Research Question and/or Hypothesis Statement

Research questions and/or hypotheses statements are more specific than the broad research purpose and problem statement. This allows the problem to be researchable. Well-written questions/hypotheses are critical for guiding the rest of the research study. They guide the design; identify what is being studied; who is being studied; and what the researcher thinks will be the results or outcome of the study. For now, this is enough about research questions and hypotheses.

Selecting a Theoretical Framework or Creating a Conceptual Framework

A study's framework may have either a theoretical framework or a conceptual framework. A theoretical framework is more formalized and abstract than a conceptual framework. However, a theoretical framework is stronger in design and provides a firmer foundation to support the study.

Often, a study does not include a theoretical framework. When this is the case, then what you have is a conceptual framework, that is, the argument is made for doing the study by using prior research to present proposed conceptual relationships.

Selecting the Best Design

The study design is a road map or blue print for doing the study. There are numerous types of designs, but the two main categories of designs are quantitative and qualitative. Quantitative designs are more formal and objective than qualitative designs. The data generated from quantitative designs are numbers, whereas for qualitative research, the data are left in words/narrative. In general, if you are interested in describing, explaining, or predicting phenomena of interest, and you want to take those findings and generalize beyond the study sample, then your best choice is a quantitative design. However, if you are more interested in the holistic perspective, which requires depth and richness of data collection, and you are not interested in generalizing your findings beyond the study sample, then a qualitative design would be the best choice. For example, Creedon's (2006) study on hand washing compliance used a quantitative design (quasi-experimental). The researchers were primarily interested in testing hand hygiene intervention with a group of healthcare workers on hand washing compliance. The goal of this study was to take the findings and generalize to at least all other healthcare workers within the study organization. They were not interested in the feelings and attitudes of the workers as much as they were in just testing whether their intervention increased hand washing within their facility.

Identification of the Sample

Once the researcher has identified the research question, has critically reviewed the related literature, and has tentatively decided on a design, they must then choose the population and the study sample. A population refers to the group under study. This is the group for whom the study findings can be generalized. The sample is the group of participants taken from the study population that are included in the actual research study.

Deciding on Data Collection Issues

Data collection decisions include the study population and sample, gaining access to the population, getting all of the approvals needed to do the study, deciding on what data will be collected to answer the research questions, and who, where, and how long it will be collected. Selection of study instruments to measure the outcomes of the study is also a critical step in data collection.

Feasibility Issues

Conducting research involves many resources from money, to time, to expertise of the research team. A proposed budget addresses these costs and provides potential funding organizations/agencies with information to make an informed decision as to their monetary commitment.

Analyzing the Data and Determining Findings

The focus of this step of the research process is to make some sense of the collected data. Data collected from quantitative studies result in numbers so that statistical analyses can be performed to answer the research questions. For qualitative studies, data are analyzed from narrative, usually by identifying themes across participants.

Dissemination of Findings

Research is useless no matter how good it is if no one knows about it. Findings must be communicated, especially if they have the potential to impact nursing practice and patient care. Common forums for communication of study findings include publication in various nursing journals, oral and poster presentations at professional meetings/conferences, and/or in the workplace. Now that a small introduction to nursing research and the research process has been discussed, we can move on to some different but similar concepts in nursing research.

WHAT IS RESEARCH UTILIZATION?

Research utilization is just that, applying research to nursing practice. During the late 1970s and early 1980s, research utilization became a popular term primarily because of two major projects. The WICHE (Western Interstate Commission for Higher Education) and CURN (Conduct and Use of Research in Nursing) projects played a critical role in increasing nursing research activities, particularly the application of nursing research findings to practice (Krueger et al., 1978; Horsley, 1981, 1982). These projects represented the first large-scale attempts to reduce the gap between nursing research and practice.

The WICHE was a 6-year project funded by the US Department of Health, Education, and Welfare. Part III of the final report was devoted to research utilization. The implications of this project were two-fold for research utilization; nurses must have the skills to analyze research for application to practice, and nurse researchers need to write implications for nursing practice into their research publications. These implications should be written in as simplified a manner as possible and should include more clinical research.

The CURN, a 5-year project sponsored by the Michigan State Nurses' Association, had as goals to stimulate the conduct of research in clinical settings and to help nurses find ways to apply research findings to their practice. The project culminated in nine volumes (Horsley, 1981, 1982) focusing on specific clinical areas such as pain, decubitus ulcers, pre- and postoperative teaching, and closed urinary drainage systems. The impetus of the work was to make research more relevant to the bedside so that practicing nurses would see its relevance.

Research utilization, as proposed by these two projects, included the idea of a systematic process completed by a research utilization committee within the organization. The committee members would divide the work needed to propose a practice change and would act as change agents for that change within the organization. Steps of this research utilization process included the following:

- Identification of the clinical problem
- Gathering information from completed research studies that add knowledge regarding the problem
- A critical evaluation of the research
- Relevance of the research to the practice setting and the patient population
- Transforming the knowledge into actions
- Definition of patient outcomes
- Education and training needed for change
- Evaluation and follow-up of the new practice protocol with modification as needed

From these steps you can see many similarities between research utilization and the nursing process. First, problem identification and support through the assessment of research studies occurs. Current research provides possible solutions to the problem. A plan is developed along with goals. Then, implementation and evaluation of the new practice change occurs with modification as needed. Now, let us discuss a term that is popular to use today, evidence-based nursing practice (EBNP).

WHAT IS EVIDENCE-BASED NURSING PRACTICE?

One of the broadest definitions is offered by Greenberg and Pyle (2004), which is "Evidence-based practice is the use of evidence to support decision making in health care." Many would argue that evidence-based practice (EBP) has emerged out of the evidence-based medicine (EBM) movement that has existed for over 2 decades. The practice of EBM involves integrating individual clinical expertise with the best available evidence from research studies (Sackett et al., 1996). The goal of EBM is to standardize clinicians' practices, eliminating worst practices and supporting best practices, thereby reducing costs and improving quality (Tanner, 1999). As you can see, the emphasis on EBM is on the clinicians' practice and the impact of empirical research on that practice.

Evidence-based practice has a much broader context and includes many forms of evidence, not just empirical research studies. EBP definitions are varied, but all include evidence from three broad areas; empirical studies, other forms of published evidence (e.g., review articles, clinical pathways, protocols), available clinical expertise and resources, and patient preferences/nuisances. Melnyk and Fineout-Overholt (2005) define EBP as a problem-solving approach using current best evidence to answer a clinical question incorporating one's own clinical expertise and patient values and preferences. I would argue that a better term to differentiate the uniqueness of nursing practice from other disciplines would be evidence-based nursing practice (EBNP).

Even though empirical research is critical to provide the support for nursing practice, other forms of evidence can be equally important in nursing. For example, nursing practice has always emphasized the involvement of the patient in their care. However, only empirical research and the clinicians' expertise are included in the definition of EBM. Published evidence can also come in many forms other than empirical studies. Other forms of evidence such as clinical pathways, protocols, practice guidelines, and review articles also play a critical role in comprising the total evidence in EBNP. Application to the individual patient occurs by combining all of this evidence (empirical studies, nonempirical published evidence, and clinical expertise) with patient preferences, values, and uniqueness.

EBNP projects can include any identified clinical problem. Some of the more developed problem areas in nursing include pressure ulcers; falls; hospital-acquired infections; ventilator-acquired pneumonia; the impact of rapid response teams and hourly rounding in reducing adverse events such as cardiac arrest; the impact of preoperative hair removal on surgical site infection; and patency in peripheral intermittent intravenous devices, just to name a few. Much of this book is devoted to learning how to participate in EBNP as painlessly as possible, but for now, this is a large enough dose of what EBNP is all about and why it is important to you as a nurse and for your patients.

COMPARING RESEARCH AND EVIDENCE-BASED PRACTICE

Many of the terms discussed up to now (e.g., nursing research process, research utilization, evidence-based nursing practice) can be confusing, especially when you attempt to discern the similarities and the differences between

Table 1-1 Comparison of Nursing Research Process, Research Utilization, and Evidence-Based Nursing Practice

Nursing research process	Research utilization	Evidence-based nursing practice
Problem identification	Clinical problem identification	Clinical problem identification
Conducting research	Using research already conducted to solve problem	Using research already conducted
Following steps of the research process	Following steps of the research utilization process	Synthesizing all of the evidence and integrating with expert opinion and patient input
Findings usually not immediately applicable—needs to be translated to practice through research utilization or EBNP	Findings usually applied at the organizational level	Findings usually applied at the bedside and tailored to the individual patient

them. What makes this even more confusing is that there is ambiguity in the literature about definitions and application to practice. To simplify things, refer to **Table 1-1** for defining characteristics of each. As you can see by this table, there are ways to discriminate between these terms. For example, *nursing research* is the actual participation or conduct of empirical research studies, whereas *research utilization* is the critical examination and application of research findings (already completed) to solve a clinical practice problem. Lastly, EBNP is the use of many forms of evidence (including but not limited to empirical studies) along with clinical expertise available and patient preferences to solve an identified clinical practice problem and to tailor it to the individual patient. Therefore, EBNP picks up where research utilization leaves off by adding other forms of evidence and expert opinion as well as the patient's individual needs and values.

DEBUNKING THE MYTHS

"I won't ever use nursing research in my practice."

Evidence from research is one of the ingredients in evidence-based nursing practice (EBNP). EBNP is performing patient care that is supported by the evidence. This evidence can come from many sources, one of which is actual research studies. You need to ask yourself, "How can I ensure that I am providing quality patient care without having evidence to support the care provided?" Isn't that what nursing is all about; that is, providing excellent care to your patients so that they may achieve optimum outcomes? Are we not ethically bound as a profession to make the most positive impact we can in the lives of our patients? Nursing research is an important tool for gathering evidence to improve practice. Even from Nightingale's day, we knew hand washing reduced infection rates and improved healing times. This was before germ theory and the research to support why it was developed. Today, we can base this practice on research. A quick search in the cumulative index of the nursing and allied health database (CINAHL) generated 78 research-based articles ranging from hospital (Chan, Chung, & Wong, 2008) to community-based settings (Tousman et al., 2007; White, Kolble, Carlson, & Lipson, 2005) and focusing on healthcare workers (Creedon, 2006) and students (Celik & Kocasli, 2008) as well as non-healthcare workers alike (Duncan & Dealey, 2007).

An ongoing clinical issue since peripheral intermitted intravenous devices were popular (1970s) is determining the best way to maintain patency. Initially (1970s to early 1990s), the recommended policy was the SASH method (Saline, Administration of Medication, Saline, Heparin) (Kotter, 1996) to ensure patency. This procedure included flushing the device with saline, administering the medication, flushing again with normal saline, and then lastly, flushing the device with heparinized saline. Potential for contamination increased with having to access the device four different times with different syringes/needles. Through subsequent research, it has now been shown that using heparin in even small doses could cause many side-effects such as hemorrhage, allergic reactions, interactions with other medications the patient may be taking, and pain at the site (Gamby & Bennett, 1995). More recently, a review and appraisal of the evidence available on this topic revealed that heparin solution is no more effective than saline alone in maintaining patency, preventing phlebitis, and increasing duration in peripheral devices. Results of the review suggest that since the use of heparin has the potential to cause so many side-effects and complications, normal saline should be the solution of choice as it contributes to patients' safety and cost savings (Mitsiou-Tzortzi & Koutelekos, 2008).

Implementing rapid response teams within the hospital setting is another example of putting evidence into practice. Melnyk (2007) describes the latest evidence on hourly rounding and rapid response teams in decreasing adverse events in hospitals. Four of the most current research articles are summarized along with an evaluative commentary by the author. Compelling evidence from these articles suggests that hourly rounding may increase patient satisfaction and decrease falls. Evidence from research on the effects of rapid response teams support the theory that they may lead to a reduction in cardiac arrests by the early identification and treatment of a deteriorating condition of a patient. As you will learn in this book, research is not the only form of evidence needed to provide quality patient care, but it is one core component of that evidence.

"Nursing research is only for graduate-prepared nurses."

Performing evidence-based nursing practice is an expectation for BSN-prepared nurses. This includes finding appropriate measures of evidence, reading and evaluating research and available protocols and guidelines, being an effective communicator so that clinical expertise can be determined, and then synthesizing across all forms of evidence. Graduate-level prepared nurses may be the ones leading the conduct of research studies, but registered nurses of any rank may be and should be encouraged to be part of the process. In fact, the bedside/staff nurse is in a premier position to identify clinical issues/problems and participate in evidence-based nursing practice activities from the beginning. Bedside nurses have a wealth of knowledge and ideas for nursing research because they have first-hand experience with current issues/problems in direct patient care and on how practice can be safe, appropriate, and cost effective. As you can see from my prior examples, it is at the bedside where research/evidence translates into practice and the real world of nursing.

"I won't have to know anything about research unless I work in a Magnet hospital."

As already mentioned, no matter what type of organization you are in, potential employers are expecting nurses to know the basics of evidence-based nursing practice. Magnet hospitals just have a higher expectation regarding the use of EBP in their organizations. The Magnet idea, originally created in 1983, includes the 14 forces of magnetism that complete the essential elements of excellence in nursing and the provision of quality care. However, it has only been within the last 5 years that its growth has really taken off, with over 250 hospitals currently recognized as Magnet hospitals (Morgan, 2007).

The overarching goal of a Magnet program is to create a culture that values excellence in nursing care and demonstrates an ability to attract and retain professional nurses. Evidence supports that achieving Magnet recognition results in higher nurse satisfaction and a positive work environment. One of the forces of magnetism specifically addresses research and evidence-based practice as a way to improve quality patient care. This description states that nurses are involved at every level of the organization in integrating research and evidence-based practice into clinical and operational processes, taking into consideration organizational and community resources (Morgan, 2007).

"The only part of a research article that I need to understand is the discussion and findings section."

All research is flawed. If research were flawless, then there would be no need for you to take a research class or read this book. You could just look at the findings and discussion and then base your practice on those suggestions. Real people are the participants in applied nursing research, not laboratory rats. These real people have lives beyond the healthcare setting and live in noninstitutionalized communities where we cannot control everything. Because of this, every research study has its strengths and its limitations. You as a nurse will need to know how to discern these strengths and limitations and decide whether the evidence can be applied to the clinical problem/issue that you have identified. As you move forward within this book, you will find important discussions on how to analyze research studies. However, it is the goal of this book to keep it as "user friendly" as possible by including only the essential ingredients. Many other nursing research textbooks are available for you to read if you want to delve deeper into any of the content areas presented here.

OVERCOMING THE BARRIERS

Facing Your Fears

Fear: "It's too much like math and statistics!"

Solution: Try reframing this common comparison between research and math and statistics.

Many people are fearful of courses such as math and statistics and view research as being very similar. The automatic barriers go up and the lack of self-confidence sets you up for failure before you even begin. Yes, it is a different way of looking at issues/problems, and it does require some basic knowledge of research language; however, it is not rocket science! You can learn how to do it. You just need to tell yourself that it is like any other skill you have had to learn in nursing school. You just need a little time to learn the process by watching the experts and taking time to practice your new skill.

Do you remember when you learned how to take a blood pressure? You did not have a clue at the beginning. Nevertheless, with some instruction, demonstration, and practice time, you were able to perfect that skill. You first have a beginning skill level where you know the procedure but you have to think of it in discrete mechanical steps. However, the more you do, the better you are at it. The old saying that "practice makes perfect" is very true with nursing skills. That also includes reading and analyzing research and developing evidence-based practice changes. It means using the process every day. When you are in the clinical area, continually ask yourself and others why a skill, procedure, or treatment is done that way. Beware of answers such as "we have always done it that way" or "because the administration wants it that way" or the "physician ordered it that way" or "because it works."

Math and statistics are full of steps/processes to get to the answer. Nursing research and EBNP are no different. There are steps to follow. In the chapters to follow, you will be guided through these steps as painlessly as possible.

Fear: "It is just too overwhelming to learn and do especially when I already have so much to do!"

Solution: Try breaking it down into smaller, more manageable pieces.

Have you ever heard the saying, "Don't make a mountain out of a molehill"? It is easy to view EBNP as a mountain. However, what if we take that mountain and break it down into several molehills? Each molehill can represent a step of the process. One molehill could represent evidence from research studies. Another one could represent other forms of evidence such as published guidelines/protocols. Then, the next one could represent clinical expertise. Then another one could represent patient preferences/uniqueness. Then, each of these molehills can be broken down into even smaller hills. Are you getting the idea?

Fear: "I just don't have the knowledge or skill!"

Solution: Read this book and practice, practice, practice!

Evidence-based nursing practice is not done is isolation. You have access to resources as a nursing student and as a practicing nurse. People such as librarians, advanced practice nurses, peers, faculty from surrounding universities, and nurse educators are just a few resources to consult. Databases and websites also provide wonderful resources for EBP protocols and synthesis of research. Refer to **Table 1-2** for some examples of these resources. Even though we may think it is just a marketing tool, Nike may have been more right than wrong with their "Just do it" approach. Do not think about all of the reasons you can come up with to prevent you from doing EBNP. We can easily talk ourselves out of any activity that we just really do not want to do or are not sure about. However, if we went into nursing for the right reasons, using EBNP is not negotiable. We have lives in our hands that need the best possible care given the evidence available. We just need to do it!

Table 1-2   Suggested Online Resources for Evidence-Based Nursing Practice

Site/Link	Comment
USPSTF-AHRQ http://www.ahrq.gov/clinic/serfiles.htm	Evidence synthesis and systematic reviews
The Cochrane Library http://www3.interscience.wiley.com/cgi-bin/mrwhome/106568753/HOME	The Cochrane Collaboration prepares, maintains and disseminates systematic reviews of healthcare interventions focusing primarily on systematic reviews of controlled trials of therapeutic interventions. The Cochrane Database of Systematic Reviews (CDSR) includes full text of regularly updated systematic reviews of the effects of health care. The Database of Abstracts of Reviews of Effectiveness (DARE) identifies the best quality systematic reviews. DARE complements the CDSR by offering a selection of quality assessed reviews in those subjects where there is currently no Cochrane review.
The Joanna Briggs Institute for EBP and Midwifery http://www.joannabriggs.edu.au/sysmenu.html	Provides access to some best practice sheets, systematic reviews, and most executive summaries and protocols.
The Sarah Cole Hirsh Institute for Best Nursing Practices Based on Evidence http://fpb.case.edu/Centers/Hirsh/	Affiliated with the Frances Payne Bolton School of Nursing at Case Western Reserve. Systematic reviews are published in the Open Access publication "Online Journal of Issues in Nursing."
National Quality Measures Clearinghouse http://www.qualitymeasures.ahrq.gov	Sponsored by AHRQ to promote widespread access to quality measures by the healthcare community and other interested individuals. Key components include: structured, standardized abstracts (summaries) containing information about measures and their development; a utility for comparing attributes of two or more quality measures in a side-by-side comparison; links to full-text quality measures (when available) and/or ordering details for the full measure.

Learning the Language

Comparison to a Foreign Language

When you started nursing school, you had to learn nursing terminology. Now, you have to learn another language, the nursing research language. Embedded in this language is statistics, hard enough to learn on its own. No wonder nurses and students are resistant to learning how to critically appraise nursing research and participate in EBNP.

Translation into Everyday Language

Is it research, is it research utilization, or is it evidence-based nursing practice? This is like saying, "A nurse is a nurse is a nurse." These terms, often used interchangeably, are not the same. Research refers to the scientific process of conducting research. Research utilization is just that, using research. It could be viewed as the early beginnings of what is now called EBNP. These terms were discussed earlier in this chapter.

When the Going Gets Tough

The Tough Get Going

It will be difficult to take the time needed to ensure your practice is based on the evidence. Particularly until this becomes a habit, it will be easy to find a million excuses for not doing it. Instead of succumbing to this temptation, remind yourself again why you should and will continue to have an evidence-based nursing practice. Try to surround yourself with others (e.g., nursing students, staff, administrators) who feel the same way. Lead and support activities that facilitate EBNP. Activities such as forming a journal club; having an article of the week/month on the floor or in nursing student areas for all to share and discuss; setting up a reward system whereby a student/nurse can receive a reward if they participate in certain ways (e.g., serving on EBNP committees, student groups, journal clubs, participating in research).

The Tough Ask for Help

It is important to surround yourself with others who share the same desire and goals to use EBNP in their careers. Like most other activities worth doing, EBNP is difficult if not impossible to do alone. Even when all of the needed evidence is collected and synthesized, other key players will need to be involved (preferably from the beginning) so that implementation of the practice change can be successful. These key players/stakeholders need to be identified early on in the process and may include individuals such as the patient and/or family members themselves, the nurses involved in that patient's care, administrative staff, nurse researchers and/or nursing professors, and clinical experts for that area of concern.

For EBNP to work, a level of organizational support and culture must be present. Along with this support, the infrastructure to participate in these activities must also be present. Houser (2008) lists several organizational factors that create barriers. They include lack of authority for clinicians to make practice changes, lack of support from peers, demanding workloads, and lack of administrative support or incentives. Stetler (2003) states for EBP to work, that it must be part of normal daily business and built into regular work hours to facilitate participation.

The Tough Never Give Up

Passion and persistence is the answer more times than not to any frustrations that you may encounter on the path to EBNP. As already mentioned, surround yourself with others of like mind and passion. There is power in numbers, and as the resistant ones start to see the positive impact on patient care and nursing practice, they too will want to participate. Change, even positive change, causes resistance to a certain degree. Nevertheless, as the benefits and positive outcomes start to outweigh the barriers and negative perspectives, this resistance will lessen and nurses/students will start to embrace the process.

THE BIG "SO WHAT?"

- Nursing research is important to answer questions about nursing practice.
- Nursing research is conducting actual research studies, whereas research utilization and EBNP are using research already completed.
- EBNP is much broader and more complex than research utilization but is critical for applying research to practice at the bedside.
- EBNP involves using current best evidence to answer clinical questions incorporating available clinical expertise and patient values and preferences.
- Nurses are expected to know how to do EBNP in the workplace.
- Knowing how to do EBNP is an expectation for all professional nurses, not a nice-to-know item.
- Use of EBNP at the bedside is the best approach for providing quality patient care and ensuring optimum outcomes.
- Reading and critically consuming research is a required component of EBNP.
- Reduce resistance to learning and doing EBNP with the "Just do it" approach.
- Breaking EBNP into smaller parts will make it easier to learn and do.
- Practice, practice, practice . . .
- Never give up.

REFERENCES

Celik, S., & Kocasli, S. (2008). Hygienic hand washing among students in Turkey. *Applied Nursing Research, 21,* 207–211.

Chan, E., Chung, J., & Wong, T. (2008). Learning from the severe acute respiratory syndrome (SARS) epidemic. *Journal of Clinical Nursing, 17,* 1023–1034.

Creedon, D. (2006). Healthcare workers' hand decontamination practices: An Irish study. *Clinical Research, 15,* 6–26.

Duncan, C., & Dealey, C. (2007). Hand hygiene. Patient's feelings about hand washing, MRSA status and patient information. *British Journal of Nursing, 16,* 34–38.

Gamby, A., & Bennett, J. (1995). A feasibility study of the non-heparinised 0.9% sodium chloride for transduced arterial and venous lines. *Intensive and Critical Care Nursing, 11,* 148–150.

Greenberg, M., & Pyle, B. (2004). Achieving evidence-based nursing practice in ambulatory care. *Viewpoint, 26, 1,* 8–12.

Horsley, J. (1981, 1982). *Using research to improve nursing practice* (Series of Clinical Protocols, 9 vols.). New York, NY: Grune and Stratton.

Houser, J. (2008). *Nursing research: Reading, using, and creating evidence.* Sudbury, MA: Jones and Bartlett.

Kotter, R. (1996). Heparin vs saline for intermittent intravenous device maintenance in neonates. *Neonatal Network, 15,* 43–47.

Krueger, J. C., Nelson, A. H., & Wolanin, M. O. (1978). *Nursing research: Development, collaboration, and utilization.* Germantown, MD: Aspen.

Melnyk, B., & Fineout-Overholt, E. (2005). *Evidence-based practice in nursing and healthcare: A guide to best practice.* Philadelphia, PA: Lippincott, Williams, & Wilkins.

Melnyk, B. (2007). The latest evidence on hourly rounding and rapid response teams in decreasing adverse events in hospitals. *Worldviews on Evidence-Based Nursing,* 4th quarter, 220–223.

Mitsiou-Tzortzi, M., & Koutelekos, I. (2008). Finding the evidence for keeping the patency in peripheral intermittent intravenous devices. *Health Science Journal, 2,* 121–128.

Morgan, S. (2007). *The forces of magnetism: Core characteristics to achieve magnet recognition.* Retrieved from http://www.medscape.com/viewarticle/562944.

Sackett, D., Rosenberg, W., Muir Gray, J., Haynes, R., & Richardson, W. (1996). Evidence-based medicine: What it is and what it isn't. *British Medical Journal, 312,* 71–72.

Stetler, C. (2003). Role of the organization in translating research into evidence-based practice. *Outcomes Management, 7,* 97–103.

Tanner, C. (1999). Evidence-based nursing practice: Why is it important? *AACN Clinical Issues: Advanced Practice in Acute and Critical Care, 12,* 469–476.

Tousman, S., Arnold, D., Helland, W., Roth, R., Heshelman, N., Casteneda, O., et al. (2007). Evaluation of a hand washing program for second graders. *Journal of School Nursing, 23,* 342–348.

White, C., Kolble, R., Carlson, R., & Lipson, N. (2005). The impact of a health campaign on hand hygiene and upper respiratory illness among college students living in residence halls. *Journal of American College Health, 53,* 175–181.

CHAPTER 2

The Quantitative Research Process

The research process is the series of steps typically followed by a researcher in the conduct of a research study. The main steps of the research process are the problem statement, literature review, theoretical/conceptual framework, research questions/hypotheses, research design, sample, data collection, data analysis, findings/recommendations, strengths/limitations, and dissemination of study findings.

PROBLEM STATEMENT

As mentioned in Chapter 1, identification of the problem is the first step and can be one of the most difficult steps. The difficulty usually comes because it can be very challenging to refine the problem statement enough so that it is research-able. Usually, the researcher moves from a broad area of interest such as "health promotion" to a more specific problem such as compliance with physical activity for Mexican-American adults. Health promotion is too broad to research without narrowing it down more. Ask yourself, "What particular area of health promotion am I interested in?" Is it physical activity, nutrition, stress reduction, health protection measures, etc.? What if I am interested in physical activity? Again, the area of physical activity is also too broad. Is it its relationship to obesity and morbidity? Is it the physiologic or psychological benefits of physical activity? On the other hand, is it motivational and behavioral issues related to physical activity? If it is exercise motivation, then you also have to think about what population you are interested in working with. Is it children, teenagers, adults, or older adults? Is it a particular culture or ethnicity? Is it the elite athlete or the everyday "Joe" who struggles with maintaining an exercise program? Now, you can see why this first step can be one of the most difficult.

LITERATURE REVIEW

Once the researcher has developed the problem statement, they can proceed with the literature review. To assess what is known and what is not known about a particular problem, a review of the literature is necessary. Information from the literature review can guide the researcher regarding what types of studies to conduct. The review guides the researcher as to selection of type and level of design, age group, gender, ethnicity, etc., or even if the study should be done at all depending on whether or not enough knowledge already exists to make a practice change. Reasons for doing a literature review are summarized in **Table 2-1**. Literature to support doing an actual research study primarily comes from empirical research, both from nursing and from related disciplines such as psychology or epidemiology. However, other sources of support may include guidelines, opinion articles, and review articles.

Electronic databases are an excellent way to begin the literature review. Libraries at universities and many hospitals purchase subscriptions through various vendors such as Ovid, EBSCOhost, Proquest, Gale powersearch, and

---

Table 2-1   Reasons for Doing a Literature Review

1. Helps to determine what has already been done that relates to the problem of interest.
2. Helps to develop a framework for the problem.
3. Provides ideas about the kinds of studies that need to be done. Previous researchers often make suggestions regarding problems that need further investigation.
4. Points out research strategies, specific procedures, and information regarding measurement instruments that have been found to be productive as well as nonproductive for the problem. Therefore, it helps the researcher to profit from and build on the experiences of others.
5. Helps the researcher to interpret the results of the study after it has been conducted by guiding the discussion of the findings in terms of agreement or nonagreement with other studies.
6. Helps the researcher develop an analytic and critical appraisal of the important and recent substantive and methodological developments in the researcher's area of interest. The researcher should explain how their study will refine, revise, or extend what is now known about the topic of interest.
7. Informs and lends support to the researcher's assumptions, operational definitions, and methodological procedures by demonstrating that the study to be done has profited from the prior research.
8. Provides a sense of context and a sense of history.

PubMed. Several of these include MEDLINE, a huge index of medical journal articles, and CINAHL, an index of articles in nursing and allied health journals. Librarians at local universities or at your own institution can be invaluable in pointing you in the right direction. A qualified librarian can assist you in deciding which electronic databases to select and what search terms to use that will yield the best results. They can also assist you with finding other types of resources both electronically and in other formats that may contribute evidence to your EBNP project. Some of the most common nursing research journals include *Nursing Research, Advances in Nursing Science, Applied Nursing Research, Clinical Nursing Research, Journal of Advanced Scholarship, Journal of Research in Nursing and Health, Journal of Nursing Measurement, Western Journal of Nursing Research, and International Journal of Nursing Studies*. You can access all of these journals through the online databases described earlier in this paragraph.

Another source of literature to examine is the references from an article you found from the electronic search. You may find some very relevant literature in relation to the problem and useful methodologies such as measurement tools that would be helpful in a study's proposal. A literature review is not just a summary of each article but is a critical analysis of each article. Further, the investigator must show how it contributes to the current proposed study.

The scope of the literature review may include the following major types of literature:

- Empirical nursing research studies
- Empirical studies from related disciplines (psychology, sociology, epidemiology, anthropology, etc.)
- Literature to support your theoretical/conceptual framework—relevant specialty nursing literature (*Public Health Nursing, Heart and Lung, Maternal Child Nursing*, etc.)
- Methodological literature to support selection of valid and reliable data collection instruments

Ultimately, the literature review should demonstrate why the study was done either by adding new scientific knowledge, validating existing knowledge, or filling in knowledge gaps.

THEORETICAL/CONCEPTUAL FRAMEWORK

A theory is a set of integrated concepts and proposed relationship statements between concepts. A nursing theory is a worldview that explains phenomena important to nursing practice. Common phenomena in nursing theories include client/person, environment, and nursing. Theory is abstract rather than concrete because it is an expression of the theorist's ideas regarding phenomena. Quantitative research is used for theory testing, whereas qualitative research can be used to generate theories.

Concepts and constructs are the building blocks of theory. A concept is a term that describes a phenomenon abstractly. Constructs are even more abstract than concepts and tend to be unique to the theory. A theory of motivation called reversal theory (Apter, 1989) identifies several constructs that are unique to the theory. For example, meta-motivational state is a term that is unique to reversal theory. Four pairs of meta-motivational states included in the theory are telic/paratelic, mastery/sympathy, autic/alloic, negativistic/ conformist states. As you can see, these terms are theory specific and lose meaning outside of the theory. The theory could be applied to something practical such as motivation for physical activity. Exercise motivation would be an example of a concept and could be measured by an exercise motivation questionnaire developed using reversal theory constructs. For this example, a relational statement between concepts/constructs could be, "Higher exercise motivation leads to higher levels of physical activity." The concepts here would be exercise motivation and physical activity.

The quantitative hand washing compliance study done by Creedon (2006) depicts one example of research used to test theory. The researcher selected the PRECEDE health education theory to develop the study's intervention. In the PRECEDE theory, the concept of behavior is dependent on factors that predispose (attitudes, beliefs, knowledge), enable (access), and reinforce (feedback) to promote a particular behavior. The interventional program aimed to predispose, enable, and reinforce healthcare workers' compliance with hand-hygiene guidelines. Healthcare workers received an educational handout and poster campaign that predisposed them to comply with hand-hygiene guidelines. An alcohol hand rub served as the enabler for hand cleaning. Feedback and results from the pretest reinforced hand washing-hygiene behavior.

Carron and Cumbie (2005) provides an example of how qualitative research is used to develop theory. The study used a grounded theory approach to develop a nursing model for the implementation of spiritual care in adult primary healthcare settings by advanced practice nurses. This qualitative approach was used to examine the manner in which patients, advanced practice nurses, Benedictine nuns, spiritual educators, and community spiritual leaders perceive spirituality and spiritual health care. This model was developed to guide spiritual care interventions by healthcare providers.

Many times a research study lacks a theoretical framework. In this case, what you have is a conceptual framework. A conceptual framework is a clearly organized and presented literature review that explicitly identifies the concepts and the hypothesized relationships among those concepts. The concepts are then defined both conceptually and concretely so that the reader can fully understand why one variable is expected to cause the other. Unfortunately, in many studies, the framework remains vague and unclear and only implicitly developed at best.

RESEARCH QUESTIONS/HYPOTHESES

The research questions/hypotheses flow from the problem statement. This is just another example of how important a good problem statement is to the overall study. Some nursing research studies may only have a problem statement, while others may have research questions and hypothesis statements. It really depends on the level of design and the research questions. For example, it is very appropriate to have only a problem statement in descriptive level research. For more rigorous designs such as quasi-experimental and experimental, formal hypothesis statements are more appropriate. For example, Creedon (2006) studied healthcare workers' compliance with hand-hygiene guidelines before and after implementation of a multifaceted hand-hygiene program. Specifically, their research questions were:

"Does a multifaceted interventional hand-hygiene program positively affect healthcare workers' compliance with hand washing guidelines in an ICU? Does a multifaceted interventional hand-hygiene program positively affect healthcare workers' attitudes, beliefs, and knowledge about hand washing guidelines?"

From these research questions, you can see that there is a proposed intervention, and that the goal of the research is to determine the effects of this intervention on hand washing compliance. Therefore, these are examples of more formalized research questions for a quasi-experimental research design.

Hypotheses are statements about predicted relationships between concepts of interest and are called variables. A variable is any factor that varies. For example, age, values, attitudes, and health status are examples of variables. Variables are categorized as either dichotomous or continuous. An example of a dichotomous variable is gender, which is either male or female. Continuous variables have a range of values and include things such as age, weight, blood pressure, and temperature.

Variables can also be categorized as independent or dependent within a hypothesis. Independent variables are the treatments or interventions that the researcher manipulates. The independent variable can stand alone and must precede the measurement of the dependent variable. The dependent variable is the outcome variable and is influenced by the independent variable. The dependent variable is what is measured as the result of the independent variable/intervention. Variables are neither inherently independent nor dependent. A variable can be an independent variable in one study and a dependent variable in another study based on the way it is stated. Hypotheses can also be categorized as either simple versus complex or directional versus nondirectional. Simple hypotheses contain only one independent variable and one dependent variable. To qualify as a complex hypothesis, there must be more than one independent and/or dependent variables. **Table 2-2** provides an analysis of several examples of hypothesis statements.

Table 2-2   Research Hypotheses Examples

<u>**Hypothesis 1:**</u>

Older patients are more at risk of experiencing a fall than younger patients.

Independent variable: age
Dependent variable: fall rate
Simple (one independent and one dependent variable), directional hypothesis (more)

<u>**Hypothesis 2:**</u>

Structured preoperative support is more effective in reducing surgical patients' perceptions of pain and requests for analgesics than structured postoperative support.

Independent variable: type of support
Dependent variable: perceptions of pain and requests for analgesics
Complex (two dependent variables), directional hypothesis (more)

<u>**Hypothesis 3:**</u>

Positive health practices are favorably affected by high self-esteem and greater amounts of social support.

Independent variable: self-esteem and social support
Dependent variable: positive health practices
Complex (two independent variables), directional (favorably)

<u>**Hypothesis 4:**</u>

Men and women will differ with respect to reported frequency and type of behaviors that could lead to the transmission of HIV.

Independent variable: gender
Dependent variable: frequency and type of risky behaviors
Complex (two dependent variables), nondirectional (differ)

CONFOUNDING/EXTRANEOUS VARIABLES

Another type of variable that is important to address is the confounding or extraneous variable. These are variables that are not of primary interest to the investigators but exist as part of the study. Since the majority of nursing research takes place in real-world community settings with human subjects and not laboratory rats, it is impossible not to have potential confounding variables within a study. The important thing is that the investigator identify what these variables are early on in the study and what attempts are being made to control for their effect. Addressing potential confounding variables is most critical in experimental designs since these require more control and rigor over the study. Strategies that a researcher can use to control for extraneous variables are to eliminate them from the study, statistically control for them, match participants in the experimental and control groups on that variable, add the variable into the study as an independent variable, and randomly select and/or assign participants into treatment groups.

The best way to control for confounding variables is to eliminate them from the study. For example, if the researcher is interested in the effects of an individualized exercise intervention on physical activity compliance in Mexican-American adults, the sample should include only Mexican-American adults. Children and other ethnicities would not be included in the study. However, this kind of control is often impossible. For example, there are several potential confounding variables in something as simple as a cookie experiment where you are comparing two different sugar cookies on taste, quality, appearance, and texture. The order of batches of cookies, type of baking sheet (shiny versus dark), cooking times, slight differences in amount of ingredients, cookie size, time of day of experiment, whether participants even like that kind of cookie or whether they had just eaten prior to experiment are all potential confounding variables. The investigator can attempt to reduce these effects by making the cookies the same as much as possible so that the only difference is the one ingredient of interest: low fat margarine versus butter. They could do the experiment at the same time of day and include those that had not just eaten. They could also include a question on the data collection instrument that asked the tasters to rate how much they liked sugar cookies and statistically test for differences.

When feasible, always use a random sample. The best way to randomize a sample is to ensure that everyone in the target population has an equal opportunity in being selected for the sample. Strategies to accomplish this will be discussed later in this chapter. When random selection is not possible, the next best thing is random assignment into treatment groups. Even though the initial sample is not randomized, random assignment into the treatment and control groups reduces the effect of confounding variables. The goal of random assignment is to ensure that equal amounts of the potential confounder are in each group, which creates a cancelling effect of the confounder across groups.

When it is not feasible to randomize or eliminate the potential confounding variable, the next choice would be to statistically control for it. Using an analysis of covariance when possible is an example of how one could statistically control for the variable. This statistical procedure is able to remove (covary) the effects of that variable from the analysis.

The investigator can match subjects in the control and experimental groups on the potential confounding variable. Matching is an arduous process that takes quite a bit of time to complete and can be difficult to do if there are unequal amounts of the variable in the sample. Because of this, elimination, randomization, or statistically controlling for the potential confounder(s) should be the preferred choices.

RESEARCH DESIGN

As discussed in Chapter 1, selection of research design depends primarily on the research question(s) asked. These questions flow from the research problem and purpose statement. For a review of the different levels of quantitative research designs, see Chapter 3. Table 3-3 presents examples on how to decide between a quantitative and qualitative design. A decision tree, located in Figure 3-1, guides the selection of quantitative design. If a qualitative approach works best to answer the question, then Table 3-5 provides major characteristics of some of the more common qualitative methodologies to guide selection.

SAMPLING

There are two main types of sampling procedures: probability and nonprobability. The main distinction between the two is that probability sampling is through random sampling techniques and nonprobability sampling is not. Probability or random sampling requires that every participant within the defined population have an equal chance of being included in the study's sample. To ensure that the sample is representative of the population, probability sampling should be done when feasible. That way, the researcher is able to generalize their study findings from the sample back to the target population. Ultimately, this is the goal of quantitative research. Two types of probability sampling are simple random sampling and stratified random sampling. With simple random sampling—use of a random numbers table or computerized random numbers table—everyone in the target population has an equal chance of selection.

Stratified random sampling involves identifying relevant strata, determining the percentage of that strata in the target population, and sampling the same amount in the sample. For example, Wilson (1993) provides an example using patients with collagen diseases. If the target population has 3% lupus, 95% arthritis, and 2% scleroderma, the same proportions should be used in the sample.

Nonprobability sampling is nonrandom sampling of participants from the overall target population. Participants are selected for the study based on things such as convenience or word of mouth. Even though it offers less chance of obtaining a representative sample, many nursing research studies involve this type of sampling. Many times nurse researchers have to settle for nonprobability sampling because of feasibility issues such as time and costs to obtain a random sample. Further, informed consent to participate in the study is required ethically to protect participants from being or feeling pressured to participate. However, this freedom to participate or to withdraw at any time limits the possibility of truly obtaining a nonbiased sample. This does not imply that this type of sampling should not be used. For qualitative research, it will be the sampling of choice since you are not interested in generalizing study findings, and your primary aim is to explore the richness and depth of experiences by participants of some phenomena of interest such as coping or pain or dying.

Convenience sampling is one of the most common forms of nonprobability sampling. It is easier to obtain a convenience sample because it allows the use of any available group of research participants. College students are frequently recruited due to ease of accessibility to researchers. Purposive sampling is popular in qualitative research. In this subjective sampling method, the investigator uses their own judgment to decide who is most representative of the study population. For example, in a study examining midlife women's attitudes toward physical activity, the authors recruited a multiethnic group of 15 midlife women (Im et al., 2008).

Another critical aspect to sampling is the sample size issue. As a researcher, you would want to obtain a large enough sample size to answer your research questions/hypotheses, but recruitment and retention of study participants cost time and money. Thus, knowing some rules of thumb to ensure an adequate sample size is useful. In general, more is better in regards to sample size, because the larger the sample size, the more representative it is of the population. You can have the best-designed study in the world, but if your sample size is not adequate, you will not get significant findings even when they do exist.

Factors to consider when analyzing sample size include how similar or different the population members are, the hypothesized strength of the relationship between factors or variables of interest, possible attrition (dropout), number of groups sampled from the population,and precision of data collection measures. The more similar a population is, the more representative the sample taken from the population will be. Increased diversity of the population will result in an increased opportunity that the sample will not be representative of the overall population. For diverse populations, a larger sample size will be required to increase representativeness.

If there is reason to believe that the treatment and control groups will be significantly different on the dependent variable (outcome measure), then a larger effect size can be anticipated, and a smaller sample size required to detect this difference. However, if there is no reason to believe this (i.e., lack of prior research), then the researcher needs to assume a small-to-moderate effect size will be present and a larger sample size will be needed to detect the hypothesized relationship between variables.

Attrition or dropouts within a study are an expected but unwelcome event. Ethically, research participants cannot be forced to join or stay in a research study. This is particularly a problem with studies that require multiple data collection points and go for an extended time (subject burden). Based on the study design and anticipated "subject burden," a certain percentage of attrition is built into the design from the beginning. For example, if you are doing a mailed out survey, you would need to mail out twice as many surveys as you expect returned, which would be the commonly accepted 50% attrition rate expected of these types of surveys.

Lastly, sample size requirements must take into account the number of groups within the study. For example, say that a researcher is interested in the impact of a hand washing intervention on healthcare workers' compliance in a hospital. They may also be interested in what types of healthcare workers are the most compliant. To answer this question, the researcher could divide the sample into nurses, physicians, and unlicensed staff and then compare compliance rates among these groups. Separating the sample into subsamples reduces the number in each group. Thus, it is important to consider this in the initial recruiting of participants.

Many nursing research studies result in nonsignificant findings. Many times this is due to the study containing too small of a sample to pick up differences or relationships between variables even when in reality they exist. This is referred to as the power of the study. In the situation described above, the statistical power of the study was too low to detect significant findings even when they were present. Power analysis is a statistical procedure that can be done preferably before the study is finished so that the researcher knows the minimum sample size that needs to be recruited to answer the research questions/ hypotheses correctly. Consumers of research can also perform power analysis after completion of the study as a way to appraise whether the study had an adequate sample size to get accurate findings or not. The statistical procedure can be done by power analysis software easily available online or by using power analysis tables found in most graduate nursing research texts and in Cohen (1988). To perform a power analysis, the first three elements listed below must be known:

1. Significance level or alpha (the acceptable norm is 0.05)
2. Effect size (unless the researcher has reason to believe otherwise, a moderate effect size is usually selected)
3. Power (the acceptable norm is 0.80)
4. Sample size (as the sample size increases, power also increases)

To test the hypotheses or research questions of a study, a cutoff point or alpha or level of significance is the probability level at which the results/differences are judged to be statistically significant between groups. As mentioned, the norm is 0.05. Significance level is also the probability of committing what is called a type I error. A significance level of 0.05 means that there is a probability of only 5 out of 100 times that the findings are due to chance alone. If a researcher makes a type I error, they are saying that there are statistically significant differences between groups on the variables of interest when there really are not.

The other type of possible error regarding decisions about hypothesis or research questions is called a type II error. A type II error is stating that there are not any differences between groups on the study's variables, when in reality there are statistically significant findings. There is a balancing act between the probability of committing a type I or type II error. As your probability of committing a type I error goes down (i.e., making your significance level even smaller such as 0.01), your probability of committing a type II error goes up. If the consequences of making a type I error are worse (e.g., treatment with life or death results), then a much more rigid level of significance is chosen (i.e., 0.01), whereas if making a type I error is not that serious, a more relaxed alpha (e.g., 0.10) may be chosen.

Effect size is the measure of how different the groups are on the dependent variable(s) within a study. If anxiety levels are measured in a group of nursing students before taking a final exam and then after the exam is over, a large difference or effect size in anxiety might be expected between the two periods. If only a small difference in anxiety level is expected, the effect size would be small. Unless there is prior research or other rationale to support differently, a medium effect size is usually chosen to conduct a power analysis.

DATA COLLECTION

Data collection decisions include the study population and sample; gaining access to the population; getting all of the approvals needed to do the study;

deciding on what data will be collected to answer the research questions; and who, where, and how long it will be collected. Selection of study instruments to measure the outcomes of the study is also a critical step in data collection. Creedon's study on hand washing identified the study population as a large (344 beds) urban hospital in Ireland. The sample was recruited from a Medical-Surgical ICU. Ethical approval was received, and the researcher herself did all of the data collection. Data was collected through a self-report questionnaire and by an observational tool. Data was collected randomly in 2-hour increments from 8 a.m. to 10 p.m. One month was allowed for collection of pretest data and the intervention. The posttest phase was collected 7 weeks after the intervention for a period of 1 month (Creedon, 2006).

Data Collection Instruments

Instruments used to collect data during a quantitative research study can range from questionnaires to rating scales, performance checklists, or very refined physiologic measures such as blood tests, vital signs, weight, etc. Data collected for quantitative studies are numerical so that the study variables can be measured. Statistics can then be applied to these numbers.

A minimum acceptable level of validity and reliability of the data collection instrument is necessary before using it in an actual research study. Validity refers to the precision and accuracy of measurement, and reliability refers to the consistency of the measurement. Validity asks the question, "Does this instrument really measure what it purports to measure?" For example, if you have an instrument that purports to measure anxiety but in reality is a measure of depression, then it is not a valid measure of anxiety. Reliability asks the question, "Does this instrument measure whatever it is measuring consistently both across subjects and within subjects with repeated measures?" Following is a discussion on the tests used to provide support for an instrument's validity and reliability.

Validity

Construct validity can be viewed as an overarching form of validity that supports that the constructs or the concepts of the study really do measure what is being purported. For example, if a researcher uses a hardiness scale, and it has construct validity, then you can have some assurance that you are actually measuring hardiness and not something else such as resilience. Content validity, predictive validity, convergent validity, divergent validity, and discriminant validity add support to this overarching construct validity.

Content validity is a systematic assessment of the content of an instrument to ensure that it represents the entire content area specified. A minimum acceptable level of content validity must be obtained before the instrument can be used in research. Content validity can be verified using the Waltz, Strickland, and Lenz (2005) two-stage process. In the first stage, each content area is outlined, and representative behaviors or attitudes are identified. In the second stage, the content is given, usually in a 1 to 4 relevancy rating scale, to a minimum of 6 experts in the content area. These individual relevancy ratings can then be tallied for agreement and a content validity index (CVI) calculated. A minimum CVI of 0.80 is needed to ensure that the instrument has content validity. Predictive validity assesses how well a score on an instrument can predict future performance. A common example is whether ACT scores predict success in college.

Convergent validity is evidence that different methods of measuring the same construct yield similar findings, whereas divergent validity is the ability to discriminate the construct from opposite concepts. For example, if a researcher wants to determine convergent validity of a new instrument designed to elicit motives for participation in physical activity, they could administer another similar well-developed instrument along with this new one. The scores on the two measures will be positively related.

For divergent validity, the newly developed instrument would be given along with a well-developed instrument measuring an opposite construct. The two measures will be negatively related for evidence of divergent validity. Convergent and divergent validity can be tested by performing a correlation between the two sets of scores on the two measures. To examine discriminant validity, the researcher could also administer an instrument that measures a similar but different construct. For example, two instruments might measure the closely related concepts of resilience and hardiness or coping and adaptation. Statistical analyses could be performed to test the ability of both instruments to discriminate between the two concepts.

Reliability

Reliability is a test of stability within an instrument and over time. Stability within an instrument, called internal validity, is evaluated by performing an alpha coefficient statistic called a Cronbach's alpha. For a new instrument, coefficient alpha should have a value of 0.70 or greater to be considered reliable. For stability over time, the most common method used is test–retest reliability. To evaluate test–retest reliability, the study participants complete the measure and then return on average 2 weeks later to take it again. Scores on the two measures should be highly correlated if the instrument has stability over time. Test–retest reliability should be 0.80 or better to be considered good. Test–retest reliability is considered the weakest form of reliability due to many issues. One issue is that many traits do change over time regardless of other factors. Further, attitudes, opinions, and/or beliefs may change just from the act of taking the test. Testing conditions might be different the second time, or a person might be sick and have that condition influence how they would respond. To help reduce these effects, retesting is done on average within 2 weeks from the initial testing.

You can have reliability without validity but not validity without reliability. You can be consistently measuring the same thing, but you may not be measuring what you think you are measuring. For example, you use a scale to measure weight of the study participants. You follow the same procedure for weighing with each participant. However, the scale has not been calibrated. You are measuring participant's weight consistently each time but with a scale that is not accurate since it has not been calibrated. Validity and reliability of your data collection instruments is critical to the overall validity and reliability of your study. If you collect data that has questionable validity and/or reliability, your study is worthless since the study results are then questionable.

DATA ANALYSIS

The focus of this step of the research process is to make some sense of the collected data. Data collected from quantitative studies result in numbers so that statistical analyses can be performed to answer the research questions. For qualitative studies, data is analyzed from narrative, usually by identifying themes across participants.

In a quantitative design, once the data collection is complete, statistical analyses are used to answer the research questions. Let us revisit the research questions given earlier in this chapter. Specifically, the research questions were:

"Does a multifaceted interventional hand-hygiene program positively affect healthcare workers' compliance with hand washing guidelines in an ICU? Does a multifaceted interventional hand-hygiene program positively affect healthcare workers' attitudes, beliefs, and knowledge about hand washing guidelines (Creedon, 2006)?"

These questions contain both independent and dependent variables. If you will remember from the discussion on research questions/hypotheses earlier in this chapter, the independent variable is the treatment or grouping variable, and the dependent variable is the outcome measure. Thus, the independent variable precedes the dependent variable. In the first research question above, the hand-hygiene program is the treatment or independent variable, and rate of hand washing compliance by healthcare workers is the dependent variable. In the second question, the independent variable is the same but the dependent variables are workers' attitudes, beliefs, and knowledge about hand washing guidelines. Knowledge of how variables differ is important for understanding what is being measured, and how it is being analyzed.

As discussed in Chapter 1, it is not necessary to comprehend all of the mathematical steps of the statistical procedures. What is more important, given the software and technology available to producers and consumers of research, is how to interpret the results in light of the research questions and the study design. Interpretation includes being able to discern if the most appropriate statistical tests were chosen given the research design and questions undertaken. Understand that both descriptive and inferential statistics are important to accomplish this. The next chapter will include more detail on descriptive and inferential statistics and how to examine the data analysis section of a published research study.

FINDINGS/RECOMMENDATIONS

One of the most important parts to the research process is the investigator's responsibility in synthesizing the results of the study so that recommendations, particularly related to nursing practice, are clearly stated. Due to lack of time and/or knowledge, many everyday consumers of nursing research focus only on the recommendations and ignore the rest of the study. Unfortunately, the study may have fatal flaws that the consumer did not take time to find. That is why the emphasis in this book is on critically analyzing published research studies and conducting evidence-based nursing practice. This section should provide rationale for the recommendations, including findings from the current study, and be supported in the literature by other similar findings.

STRENGTHS AND LIMITATIONS

As was stressed in Chapter 1, all research studies are flawed, which means they all have inherent strengths and limitations. It is the responsibility of the investigator to "fess up" to these limitations and to identify how to prevent them in future work. Common limitations tend to center around difficulties in obtaining a sample size that is large enough and representative of the target population. As discussed, conducting true randomized controlled trials is costly in time and money. Finding adequate numbers of clients in order to select a sample can be very difficult depending on the commitment required by the participants to participate. This is referred to as "subject burden." Multiple testing, uncomfortable data collection procedures, and a long time commitment are just a few examples of what makes it difficult to obtain an adequate sample size.

Identification of the study's strengths is also important for the researcher to include. This allows a more balanced view of the overall study rigor for the reader.

DISSEMINATION OF FINDINGS

As mentioned earlier, research is useless no matter how good it is if no one knows about it. Communication of findings is critical especially if it has the potential to impact nursing practice and patient care. The first step is finding the right audience(s) for the work. For example, a study explaining the psychometric evaluation of a new measurement tool to measure resilience would be perfect for a journal such as *Journal of Nursing Measurement*, whereas its appropriateness in clinical practice journals might be questionable since most nurse clinicians might find it quite tedious and boring. However, a different article/study using this new instrument in patient populations such as those with chronic disease would be very appropriate in practice journals. Other common forums for communication of study findings include oral and poster presentations at professional meetings/conferences and/or the workplace. Now that a small introduction to nursing research and the research process has been discussed, we can move on to quantitative data analysis.

THE BIG "SO WHAT?"

- The research process follows distinct steps that include the problem statement, literature review, theoretical framework, research questions, research design, sample, data collection, data analysis, findings/recommendations, and strengths/limitations.
- It is important that the problem statement be specific enough that it can be tested.
- Literature review provides a context and support for a study.
- A literature review is not just a summary but a critical analysis of prior research.
- If a theoretical framework is absent from a study, then what you have is a conceptual framework.
- Hypotheses are statements about predicted relationships between concepts (variables) of interest.
- Variables are neither inherently independent nor dependent.
- Strategies for controlling confounding variables include randomization, elimination, statistically controlling for them, testing them as an independent variable in the study, or matching groups on the confounder.

- Probability or random sampling is the appropriate sample for experimental designs, whereas nonprobability sampling is most appropriate for nonexperimental quantitative designs or for qualitative research studies.
- Power analysis is a statistical procedure to determine minimum sample size for a quantitative study.
- Type I error is made by the researcher when they conclude that there is statistical significance when there actually is not. Type II error is made when conclusion is made that there is no statistical significance in findings when there actually is. It is the ultimate goal of the researcher not to make either error.
- A minimum level of instrument validity and reliability are both important before using the data collection tool in a study. A minimum level of content validity and a Cronbach's alpha of at least 0.70 are critical before using the tool.
- You can have reliability without validity but not validity without reliability.
- All research studies have both strengths and limitations.
- Research is useless if it is not communicated.

REFERENCES

Carron, R., & Cumbie, S. (2005). Grounded theory research to develop a nursing model for spiritual care. *International Journal for Human Caring, 9*(2), 98.

Creedon, D. (2006). Health care workers' hand decontamination practices: An Irish study. *Clinical Research, 15,* 6–26.

Im, E. O., Chee, W., Lim, H. J., Liu, Y., & Kim, H. K. (2008). Midlife women's attitudes toward physical activity. *Journal of Obstetric, Gynecologic, & Neonatal Nursing, 37,* 203–213.

Waltz, C. F., Strickland, O. L., & Lenz, E. R. (1991). *Measurement in nursing research* (2nd ed.) Philadelphia, PA: F. A. Davis.

Wilson, H. S. (1993). *Introducing research in nursing.* Redwood City, CA: Addison-Wesley.

CHAPTER 3

Quantitative Versus Qualitative Research, or Both?

NURSING RESEARCH WORLDVIEWS

Nursing research falls within the two broad worldviews, the positivist and the naturalistic paradigms. These two worldviews have opposing assumptions about reality and view of the world. For example, in regards to reality, the positivist believes that a single reality exists that can be measured, whereas in the naturalistic paradigm, there are multiple realities that are continually changing, which make it very difficult if not impossible to measure. Other important opposing assumptions are listed in **Table 3-1**.

The two main types of research methods are quantitative and qualitative. Quantitative research aligns with the positivist paradigm, whereas qualitative research most closely aligns itself with the naturalistic paradigm. Quantitative research is a formal, objective, deductive approach to problem solving. In contrast, qualitative research is a more informal, subjective, inductive approach to problem solving. More characteristics of each are compared in **Table 3-2**. Even though quantitative research has been considered the more rigorous of the two in the past, qualitative research has gained more credibility in the science world recently. In fact, both are appropriate methods for conducting research, and each method can contribute greatly to the scientific body of knowledge. Selection of which method to use depends primarily on the research question(s) being asked. These questions flow from the research problem and purpose statement.

For example, testing a new fall prevention program within your hospital would require you to obtain a baseline fall rate before the program and then again after full implementation of the program. Statistically, you could compare rate of falls before the new program with the rate of falls after the new program. Your unit of analysis would be numbers and would lend itself to a

Table 3-1   Comparison of Major Assumptions of the Positivist and Naturalistic Paradigms

Positivist paradigm	Naturalistic paradigm
There is a single reality that can be measured.	There are multiple realities that can be studied only holistically and cannot be predicted or controlled although some level of understanding can be achieved.
The researcher and the research participant can remain independent of one other and not influence one another.	The researcher and the research participant cannot remain separate or independent. They interact and influence one another.
Findings of research can be generalized from the study sample to the larger target population.	Findings cannot be generalized beyond the study sample. Knowledge gleaned from the study is in the form of "working hypotheses."
Cause and effect relationships can be tested.	Cause and effect relationships cannot be tested since there are multiple realities that are continually changing, so it is impossible to distinguish causes from effects.
Research can be conducted objectively and value free.	Research is subjective and value bound (i.e., the researcher's own values).

Table 3-2   Characteristics of Quantitative and Qualitative Research Methodologies

Quantitative research	Qualitative research
Considered a hard science	Considered a soft science
Objective	Subjective
Deductive reasoning used to synthesize data	Inductive reasoning used to synthesize data
Focus—concise and narrow	Focus—complex and broad
Tests theory	Develops theory
Basis of knowing—cause and effect relationships	Basis of knowing—meaning, discovery
Basic element of analysis—numbers and statistical analyses	Basic element of analysis—words, narrative
Single reality that can be measured and generalized	Multiple realities that are continually changing with individual interpretation

Table 3-3   Decisions Regarding Type of Design

Research question	Unit of analysis	Goal is to generalize	Methodology
What is the impact of a learner-centered hand washing program on a group of second graders? (Tousman, et al., 2007)	Paper and pencil test resulting in hand washing knowledge scores	Yes	Quantitative
What is the effect of crossing legs on blood pressure measurement? (Keele-Smith & Price-Daniel, 2001)	Blood pressure measurements before and after crossing legs resulting in numbers	Yes	Quantitative
What are the experiences of black fathers concerning support for their wives/partners during labor? (Sengane & Cur, 2009)	Unstructured interviews with black fathers (5 supportive and 5 nonsupportive); results were left in narrative form describing themes based on nursing for the whole person theory	No	Qualitative
What is the experience of hope in women with advanced ovarian cancer? (Reb, 2007)	Semi-structured interviews with women with advanced ovarian cancer (N=20) Identified codes and categories with narrative examples	No	Qualitative

quantitative design. However, if you were interested in studying the impact of falls on patient's quality of life, you would most likely obtain that information through a personal interview. The unit of analysis would be words, and a qualitative method would be the most appropriate approach to analyze this data. **Table 3-3** depicts this strategy using sample research questions.

QUANTITATIVE DESIGNS

Four main types of quantitative designs are descriptive, correlational, quasi-experimental, and experimental. In general, choice of design is greatly influenced by the level of knowledge of the research problem. If the amount of descriptive level research is abundant over a particular problem area, then the next logical step is to do a correlational study to examine relationships between variables. If the problem area has been described and the relationships between variables tested, the next level of research would be quasi-experimental or experimental research. For example, a large amount of research exists on surgical site infections, particularly descriptive, correlational, and quasi-experimental studies. It would therefore not make sense to do another descriptive or even correlational study. Instead, conducting experimental studies by testing interventions to prevent surgical site infections would be the next step.

Matching Research Design to Research Question

Dickoff and James (1968) developed four levels of researchable questions. Each level leads to a specific quantitative research design. Then, as discussed in Chapter 1, the research design then becomes the blueprint for the rest of the study, including sampling, data collection, and analysis.

Level One

Factor-isolating questions ask, "What is this?" These questions name and describe factors or variables of interest to the researcher. Questions such as, "What factors impact the decision to participate regularly in physical activity?" or "What factors influence mother–infant bonding?" would be included in this category of questions. The most appropriate research design to answer these questions would be descriptive. Descriptive studies are designed to gain more information about characteristics of a topic of interest. Descriptive level research is most appropriate when very little research is available on the topic. Factors need to be described before they can be tested. Descriptive level research includes survey research or case study methodology. Survey research involves gathering data, usually through a written survey/questionnaire. The purpose of survey research is to describe characteristics, opinions, attitudes, or behaviors as they currently exist in a target population. A case study design explores in depth a single participant or event through detailed information. Case studies are commonly used in nursing practice to depict a particular disease or illness.

One advantage to descriptive level research is that the researcher is able to collect a large amount of data. However, even though there is breadth of data, it tends to lack depth for the sample. On the other hand, case study research provides depth and richness of data but lacks breadth since it is limited to one person or event. One important distinction of descriptive level research is that nothing is manipulated or controlled. Phenomena are studied in real-life situations. Thus, cause and effect relationships cannot be determined using this design. Data are analyzed using descriptive statistics such as frequencies, means, and percentages. A comparative descriptive design adds to the basic descriptive design by making it possible to compare two or more groups on the factors of interest. In the previous example on mother–infant bonding, a comparative descriptive study could compare mother–infant bonding to father–infant bonding. Now, you have two groups and you are comparing them on the factor of interest, infant bonding.

An example of this design is McAuliffe's (2007) study on oral hygiene. The purpose of this study was to explore and identify factors that may influence nursing students' oral hygiene practice in hospitalized patients. As you recall, factor-isolating questions ask the question "What is this?" which is what McAuliffe is doing here. Only an aim and objectives, not hypotheses, were used in this study. A survey was used to gather the student's perspectives on what they were taught versus what they practiced as it relates to oral hygiene practices. Descriptive statistics (percentages) were performed to answer their objectives. Findings indicated that there was incongruence between what the students thought they were taught and what was actually taught in the classroom. Further, students were picking up not-necessarily good habits from their nurse role models within the clinical setting.

Level Two

Factor-relating questions would be the next category of research questions and would ask, "What is happening here?" Correlational research is used to answer relational type questions such as this. However, before this question can be answered, the factors or variables have to be described by either a prior descriptive level study or synthesis of published literature. Specific factor-relating questions could include "What is the relationship between depression and suicide among teenagers?" or "What is the relationship between motivation and exercise behavior?"

An advantage to using correlational research is that this method provides an evaluation of strength and direction of relationship between variables. Correlational studies also provide for a basis for experimental studies to follow. The primary disadvantage with this design is that no conclusions can be made regarding causality, just that there is a relationship between the tested variables. Predictive studies also fit under this level, and they describe the relationship between a predictor variable(s) and the dependent variable (outcome measure).

Data from correlational studies would primarily include descriptive statistics as described above and correlations. For example, correlational analysis would test whether there is a relationship between depression and suicide among teenagers, whether it is a positive or negative relationship, and how strong that relationship is.

An example of this design is a study completed by Al-Kandari, Vidal, and Thomas (2008) examining the relationship between a health promoting lifestyle and body mass index among college students in Kuwait. The study sample included all 350 nursing students enrolled in the AND program during one semester. Walker's Health Promoting Lifestyle Questionnaire (HPLP-II) was administered to assess health promoting attitudes and behaviors. A Pearson's correlation was done to find out the relationship of the levels of enrollment with the HPLP-II and BMI. Findings included a significant positive correlation between the BMI and the level of nursing course. That is, as students progressed in their nursing courses, their BMI increased.

Level Three

Situation-relating questions ask, "What would happen if?" This is the first level of researchable questions that examines causality. These types of questions are best answered through quasi-experimental designs where the researcher is evaluating some intervention. Quasi-experimental designs are called "quasi" because they lack one of the requirements of being a true experimental design. To be considered a true experimental design, there must be a treatment, control over who gets the treatment or intervention, and randomization of the treatment into treatment and control groups. The requirement most commonly lacking is randomization of the sample.

Advantages include the ability to infer causality, which is stating that the treatment (independent variable) caused the effect in the outcome measure (dependent variable). However, the investigator cannot definitively determine causality since the sample was not randomized. Representativeness of the sample comes into question due to this lack of randomization from the target population. This type of research also provides the basis for future true experimental studies that include randomization of the sample.

Examples of specific situation-relating questions include, "Will a hand-hygiene intervention increase healthcare workers' compliance with hand hygiene?" or "Will hourly rounding decrease adverse events in hospitals?" Data analysis for these studies may include a variety of tests depending on the research question, the type of data collected, number of participant groups, and sample size.

An example of a quasi-experimental study is a hand-hygiene interventional study done by Siegel & Korniewicz (2007). The authors state that the study was conducted to investigate hand-hygiene compliance of healthcare professionals before and after the introduction of a handheld sanitizer spray. A pretest posttest quasi-experimental design was used with the pretest observations serving as the control group and the posttest observations serving as the experimental group. Participants self-selected into the study without any randomization being performed. No significant differences were found from pretest to post-test on hand-hygiene compliance.

Level Four

Situation-producing researchable questions are the highest level of inquiry, requiring the most control by the researcher. Situation-producing questions ask, "How can I make it happen?" and can include questions such as, "How can humor be used to mediate the suffering of patients in chronic pain?" or "How can an individualized exercise prescription impact exercise behavior in a group of Mexican-American adults?" Often called a randomized control trial (RCT), an experimental research design is the "gold standard" for research and evidence-based nursing practice. It provides the most convincing evidence to support the value of a treatment. To be considered experimental level research, there must be random selection and/or random assignment of subjects, control/manipulation of the treatment/intervention, and include treatment and control groups. Experimental designs are the most difficult to implement since it takes more time and money to produce a randomized sample. Also, it may not be ethically possible to withhold treatment from the control group, thus preventing a true RCT design. Further, if an experimental design is used and the investigators find that the experimental treatment is effective in producing the desired effects, the study is stopped and the treatment is given to the control group participants. **Figure 3-1** presents a decision tree on selecting the correct type of quantitative research design.

Figure 3-1   Decision tree matching research design to category of research question.

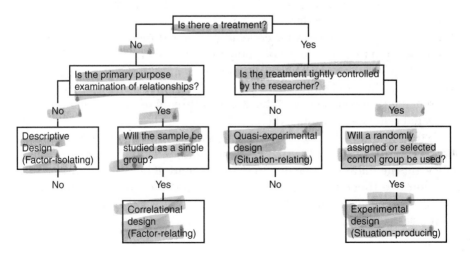

An example of an experimental study provided by Hoadley (2009) compared the effects of low- and high-fidelity simulation in learning advanced cardiac life support (ACLS). This study compared results of two ACLS classes on measures of knowledge and resuscitation skills. One of the four hypotheses was, "ACLS course participants will have significantly higher scores on the ACLS posttest when they experience computerized, high-fidelity simulation rather than instructor-led, low-fidelity simulation for resuscitation practice (Hoadley, 2009)." The theoretical framework for the study was John Dewey's experiential learning philosophy. The study sample was made up of 53 healthcare providers randomly assigned into experimental or control groups. For the sample hypothesis given above, T-tests were done to test for significant differences. No significant difference was found between the high-fidelity versus the low-fidelity modes of instruction on ACLS posttest scores.

Validity of the Research Design

Both internal and external validity are important to the overall validity of the research study. Internal validity refers to whether or not the manipulation of the independent variable really makes a significant difference on the dependent variable (Wilson, 1993). For example, an investigator may want to study the effects of an individualized exercise intervention on exercise compliance. They would want to state that the increase in exercise compliance is due to the individualized exercise intervention and not something else. Potential confounding variables, discussed in Chapter 2, can threaten internal validity. As an investigator, you want your study's findings to be a true reflection of the real world and not false findings. If the investigator makes a wrong decision regarding study findings, a type I or II error is made. Type I and II errors were introduced in Chapter 2 under the discussion on sampling. To review, a type I error is concluding that a difference exists between groups when in reality it does not. A type II error occurs when an investigator concludes that no differences exist when in reality there are significant differences. The ideal situation is not to commit either one of these errors but to make true conclusions. **Table 3-4** lists threats to internal validity and suggested remedies to reduce them.

External validity refers to the representativeness or generalizability of a study's findings. In the exercise compliance example above, we not only want the findings to be due to the intervention but we would also like to generalize those findings to a larger population. Ability to generalize findings increases as the rigor and control of the study design increases. Therefore, quasi-experimental and experimental designs offer the greatest

Table 3-4 Threats to Internal Validity with Strategies to Reduce the Threat

Threat	Remedy
History—defined as the influence of events that occur during study implementation but not part of study	Randomly select or assign into treatment and control groups to ensure the effect of history is equal in both groups.
Maturation—referring to changes that occur within the participants as a function of time	Be careful with longitudinal studies and randomly select or assign into treatment groups for the same reason as listed in #1.
Testing—referring to the effects of multiple testing; this might influence how the participant responds on successive testing	Try not to test the same participants. Build in another control group that is tested the same number of times as the treatment group so you can measure this effect.
Instrumentation—whether the instruments used for data collection were valid and reliable; can also refer to the way data collectors assign scores on the dependent variable	Keep data collectors "blind" as to which participants are assigned into what groups. Train data collectors thoroughly to collect data correctly and consistently.
Statistical regression—the tendency for subjects who initially score either very high or very low, that upon multiple testing, these scores become less extreme	Randomly select or assign participants into treatment and control groups.
Selection—referring to a tendency of types of participants to be alike (most motivated, educated, etc.)	Randomly select or assign participants into treatment and control groups.
Attrition—referring to participants that drop out of the study before completion	Give clear instructions and guidelines about required commitment for participating in the study. Collect as much demographic information as possible on these dropouts to see if they are different from the participants that continued in the study.

opportunity for generalization of study findings to a larger population. The most serious limitation of a study would only be the ability to generalize findings to the sample within the current study. Remember, the ultimate goal of quantitative research is generalizability. Thus, both internal and external validity are important to make valid conclusions and generalizations.

Before determining that a causal relationship exists between the treatment and the outcome, three conditions must exist:

1. Changes in the presumed cause must be related to changes in the presumed effect. That is, if you change the treatment, the outcome will change.
2. The presumed cause must occur before the presumed effect. That is, the treatment or intervention must come before the outcome is measured.
3. There are no plausible alternative explanations. In other words, no other factors or variables could be responsible for the outcome (Houser, 2008).

QUALITATIVE DESIGNS

Qualitative research is a systematic, subjective approach used to describe life experiences and give them meaning. Three of the most common qualitative designs that are discussed in this book are phenomenology, grounded theory, and ethnography. Table 3-2 lists some general characteristics of both quantitative and qualitative research. Additional characteristics discussed in Lincoln & Guba (1985) include:

- Natural setting
- Human as instrument
- Intuitive, felt knowledge
- Purposive sampling
- Emergent design
- Negotiated outcomes
- Tentative application
- Special criteria for trustworthiness/rigor

Natural Setting

Qualitative research is conducted in the natural setting for which the study is proposed. Based on the naturalistic worldview or paradigm, the belief is that realities cannot be understood in isolation from their contexts. For the fullest understanding, participants are recruited and studied within their natural day-to-day environment.

Human as Instrument

The researcher uses themselves and other humans as the primary data-gathering instruments, whereas in quantitative research paper and pencil or physiologic measures are more common. It is believed that the researcher influences the study findings through their interaction with the study participants, and that the human as instrument is the best one capable of grasping and evaluating the meaning of that interaction.

Intuitive, Felt Knowledge

Data collected in qualitative research is much more than the data spoken or written down by the participant. Much of the knowledge that can be gained occurs at a much more abstract, often nonverbal level. This level of knowledge is critical for really appreciating and understanding the depth of interaction between the researcher and the participants and between participants.

Purposive Sampling

Purposive sampling is a process that involves the conscious selection of certain participants for the study. Remember, the goal of qualitative research is meaning, discovery, and richness of detail of the phenomena of interest for that group of individuals experiencing that reality for that given time period. Generalizability of study findings to a larger population is not the goal as it is in quantitative research. Thus, researchers recruit participants who have the qualities they are attempting to understand. For example, if the purpose of the study were to explore what it is like to be a caregiver of a dying loved one, participants would be caregivers of dying patients.

Emergent Design

Qualitative researchers allow the research design to emerge or unfold as the study progresses rather than construct it prior to the study, as one would do with quantitative research studies. Philosophically, qualitative worldviews believe that what emerges from the data is a function of the interaction between the participant and the researcher, which cannot be determined before the study begins.

Negotiated Outcomes

Both the researcher and the participant—often through a negotiated process—determine findings from qualitative research. A process called "member checking" occurs, which involves the researcher taking the data/information that they have gleaned and reflecting this information back to the participant. Participants may or may not agree with the researcher's interpretation of the data. This process allows for some give and take between the two and a belief that the results will be a more accurate reflection of reality.

Tentative Application

Again, the goal of qualitative research is not generalizability but an understanding of a phenomenon of interest for a group of participants within a very small slice of time. Philosophically, the belief is that realities are multiple, different, and change over time and may not be duplicated anywhere else. Thus, the qualitative researcher is likely to be hesitant about trying to make broad application of findings.

Qualitative Research and Nursing Practice

Qualitative research fits very nicely with nursing practice. Nurses are experts in synthesizing data acquired through observing and listening to patients' stories about their subjective, lived experiences. As discussed in Chapter 1, understanding the meaning of a phenomenon of interest is what qualitative research is all about. For example, questions such as "understanding what it is like to live with chronic pain, living with AIDS, or living with any chronic disease" would lend themselves to qualitative research. Qualitative research is useful when the research context or the nature of the problem is poorly understood. Examples of the most common qualitative designs discussed here are phenomenology, grounded theory, and ethnography.

Phenomenology

Phenomenology is an approach to exploring people's everyday life experiences. Phenomenological researchers investigate subjective phenomena. Examples of questions asked by this type of research include, "What is this experience like?" What is the meaning of this experience or phenomena?" Phenomenology uses bracketing of preconceived values and ideas and intuitive knowledge. Participant observation is often used to collect data. This involves a combination of observing participants in a natural real-life setting and interaction of the researcher with the participant in this setting. Interviews are commonly used. Literature review is commonly done after the data has been collected to help prevent preconceived findings. Data is often presented as a clustering of themes through use of poems, pictures, and case scenarios to help describe the phenomenon. Another common characteristic of phenomenology is the use of paradigm and exemplar cases to describe the findings. Paradigm cases are whole cases that include all of the characteristics of the phenomenon, whereas exemplar cases are shorter stories that depict the phenomenon but may not include all of the characteristics.

For example, Sengane & Cur (2009) described the experience of black fathers concerning support for their wives/partners during labor. Unstructured interviews with 10 black fathers revealed both positive and negative feelings. Suggestions regarding future interventions with this population included enforcing positive feelings and removing obstacles such as lack of information, fear, and cultural factors. Tanner et al. (1993) describe the phenomenology of knowing the patient. The authors describe a paradigm case for knowing the patient as a person. They go into detail about George, a quadriplegic for many years after a motor vehicle accident who could not verbally communicate after a radical neck dissection. Participants' own words provide vivid descriptions, case scenarios, and stories.

Grounded Theory

Grounded theory, a qualitative method developed by Glaser and Strauss (1967), is an approach to theory development grounded or rooted in the data. The constant comparative method involves gathering and interpreting data simultaneously. This provides an example of the emergent design process. The design flows and changes direction based on data collection and interpretation that is occurring simultaneously. The grounded theory approach does assume the possibility of discovering fundamental patterns in life. These patterns, called basic social processes or core variables, guide the rest of data collection and analysis and are important in being able to explain and attach meaning to the study's findings.

Reb (2007) described the experience of hope in women with advanced ovarian cancer. Grounded theory approaches using focused interviews were conducted to collect data. The constant comparison method provided a means to analyze the data and the core variable that emerged from the data, which was transforming the death threat. Three phases of this process included shock (reverberating from the impact), aftershock (grasping reality), and rebuilding (living the new paradigm). Hope, linked to the core variable, was necessary for finding meaning in the experience. Support and perceived control contributed the most to hope. Hagerty et al. (1993) developed a theory of human relatedness using grounded theory. Grounded in the data through both an integrative review of the literature and through a focus group approach, states of relatedness such as connectedness and disconnectedness emerged. Social processes or core variables that contributed to movement of the individual through these states are a sense of belonging and reciprocity. Relatedness is a central idea in nursing practice and can offer a way to explain the impact of relatedness to the development of the nurse–client relationship.

Ethnography

Ethnographies focus on studying the culture of a group of people. They involve the description and interpretation of that culture's behavior. A classic phase of ethnographies is what is called "fieldwork," where the researcher becomes involved within the community and gains an "insider's perspective" through intense participant observation over an extended period (months to years). Gaining entry can be a problem particularly if it is a much-closed cultural group or the researcher comes from a different culture than the one under study. Ethnographers analyze data through rich and detailed descriptions of the culture.

Hancock and Easen (2006) examined the decision making of nurses when extubating patients following cardiac surgery. Semi-structured interviews and participant observation were used to collect data over an 18-month period.

Decision making of the nurses used other factors than the current best evidence protocol. Decision making was influenced by factors such as relationships, hierarchy, power, leadership, education, experience, and responsibility. Comparison of categories and themes between observational and interview data provided a method of data source triangulation.

As you can see by the description of each of these specific qualitative methods, there are more similarities than differences. Threats to rigor are present in each method, with some more relevant than others depending on the methodology chosen. See **Table 3-5** for a comparison of the three methodologies, giving their characteristics, purpose, and potential threats to rigor.

Special Criteria for Trustworthiness/Rigor

Trustworthiness/rigor in qualitative research is similar to validity and reliability in quantitative research. However, the conventional definitions and ways to ensure validity and reliability of a study and its findings run counter to the beliefs or worldviews of the qualitative paradigm. Internal validity fails since

Table 3-5   Characteristics of Phenomenology, Ethnography, and Grounded Theory

Phenomenology	Ethnography	Grounded Theory
Description of lived experience	Description and analysis of culture	Used for theory development
Bracketing used	Access or gaining entry to study population can be difficult	Immersed in social environment and seen through the eyes of the study participant
Data collected by interview and participant observation	Participant observation and interviews used to collect data	Data collected primarily by interviews, observation, and journal/document review
Intuit, identify, and describe phenomenon	Thick description and rich detail of data important	Constant comparison method used to collect and analyze data
Clustering of themes, paradigm versus exemplar cases	Codes to categories to clusters as a way of organizing data	Coding used to conceptualize data into patterns or concepts. Identification of core variable important for direction of rest of study

it is based on a single reality that can be measured and quantified. External validity fails because generalizability of study findings is neither the goal nor a possibility with qualitative research. Reliability fails because stability and consistency is not part of the qualitative paradigm based on researcher and study participant interaction and influence of values with each other.

Sandelowski (1986) presents an argument on how qualitative research can be rigorous without sacrificing its relevance or richness. She discusses four factors that are critical for rigor in qualitative research: truth-value, applicability, consistency, and neutrality.

Truth-value

Truth-value is similar to the internal validity that was discussed with quantitative research methods. In quantitative research, this usually involves how well threats to internal validity have been controlled (see Table 3-4). The truth-value of a qualitative study deals more with the discovery or experiences of life phenomena as they are perceived by participants. To achieve truth-value, a qualitative study must present a faithful description or interpretation of the human experience so that people having that experience can identify with it. A threat to truth-value is what Sandelowski terms "going native." "Going native" is the possibility of the researcher becoming so enmeshed with the participants that they have a difficult time separating their own experiences from that of their participants. The close relationship that often occurs between the researcher and the study participant can be viewed as both a strength and a limitation. The close bond increases trust between the two, but this closeness can also cause the researcher difficulty in separating their values and preconceived ideas from those of the participant. Bracketing, a process where the researcher mentally separates and puts "brackets" around these values, is encouraged to help decrease this threat.

Applicability

Applicability is similar to external validity in quantitative research. To ensure generalizability and representativeness, samples are randomly selected or randomly assigned into treatment groups. Power analysis procedures are used prior to beginning the study to determine how large the sample size needs to be to achieve statistical significance if present. However, sample sizes in qualitative research are generally small because of the depth of data obtained. Sandelowski (1995) shares some rules of thumb for sample sizes depending on the qualitative design used; 6 for phenomenologies, and for ethnographies and grounded theory a minimum of 30 to 50 interviews and/or observations. Sample size depends on when data saturation occurs. Reaching data saturation, which involves obtaining data until no new information emerges, is critical for obtaining applicability in qualitative research. Threats to applicability include "elite bias" and "holistic fallacy." Elite bias may occur when the most articulate, accessible, or high-status members of the group of interest volunteer to participate in the study. Holistic fallacy occurs when the researcher stops data collection prematurely before data saturation occurs, yet the researcher presents the data as complete.

Consistency

Consistency in qualitative research is similar to reliability in quantitative research. As discussed with quantitative methods, reliability is getting consistent results every time a data collection instrument is administered. In contrast, qualitative research emphasizes uniqueness of human experiences. The researcher seeks variations of these experiences. A study is consistent when another researcher can follow the "decision trail" used by the study's researcher. This is very similar to an audit done by the Internal Revenue Service (IRS). A paper trail is presented to the auditor so that they can follow your decisions on type and amount of deductions taken on your taxes.

Neutrality

Neutrality is the freedom from bias in the research process. In quantitative research, this is achieved when validity and reliability are established. In qualitative research, it occurs when truth-value, applicability, and consistency are established. Qualitative research values meaningfulness of data, which is promoted by increasing connection between the researcher and the research participant through engagement, and valuing subjectivity rather than objectivity. In general, to reduce threats to rigor, strategies such as member checking, data saturation, peer debriefing, expert panel, and triangulation may be used. Member checking and data saturation have already been discussed. Peer debriefing and expert panel involve discussing your findings and the process and decision regarding those findings with peers and experts for their feedback. Experts may come from the specific qualitative methodology used and/or from the phenomena of interest.

MIXED METHODS

A popular trend today is the planned integration of qualitative and quantitative methods within the same study. Many researchers argue that the worldviews/paradigms that underpin qualitative and quantitative research are so opposing that this cannot be done. Many others believe that using methods from both of the paradigms can be very complementary and enriching. Since each methodology has its own inherent strengths and limitations, using both may emphasize each one's strengths and minimize their limitations. One typical way to approach a mixed methods design is by doing the study in phases. For example, Keele (2009) developed a new instrument to measure exercise motives for Mexican-American adults. The process included two phases; a small qualitative portion utilizing interviews about individual motives for exercising and then a quantitative portion, which included administering the instrument developed from these interviews to a larger sample to test for instrument validity and reliability.

QUANTITATIVE VERSUS QUALITATIVE VERSUS BOTH (MIXED METHODS)?

You need all of the information presented in this chapter to be able to make correct decisions regarding choice of design. As already stated, selection of which method to use depends primarily on the research question(s) being asked. These questions flow from the research problem and purpose statement. The rest of the research process is dictated by the design choice. The simplest way to demonstrate this is by a visual depiction using decision trees.

THE BIG "SO WHAT?"

- Quantitative and qualitative research are the two main research methodologies available to researchers.
- Quantitative research parallels the positivist paradigm, and qualitative research parallels the naturalistic paradigm.
- If the goal of the research study is to generalize findings from the sample to the bigger target population, then a quantitative study is the method of choice.
- If the goal of the research study is to find meaning and understand the subjective experience of the study participants, then a qualitative study is the method of choice.
- Four of the most common quantitative designs are descriptive, correlational, quasi-experimental, and experimental.
- There are advantages and limitations with every research design.
- Causality is not examined unless the design is at a quasi-experimental or experimental level.
- External and internal validity of a study design are both important for the study's findings to be credible.
- Three of the most common qualitative research designs are phenomenology, grounded theory, and ethnography.

- Selection of research method depends primarily on the research question(s) being asked. These questions flow from the research problem and purpose statement.
- Special criteria for trustworthiness/rigor in qualitative research are truthvalue, applicability, consistency, and neutrality.

REFERENCES

Al-Kandari, F., Vidal, V., & Thomas, V. (2008). Health-promoting lifestyle and body mass index among college of nursing students in Kuwait: A correlational study. *Nursing and Health Sciences, 10*, 43–50.

Cohen, J. (1988). *Statistical power analysis for the behavioral sciences* (2nd ed.). Hillsdale, NJ: Lawrence Erlbaum Associates.

Glaser, B., & Strauss, A. (1967). *The discovery of grounded theory: Strategies for qualitative research.* New York, NY: Aldine De Groyter.

Hagerty, B., Lynch-Sauer, J., Patusky, K., & Bouwsema, M. (1993). An emerging theory of human relatedness. *Image: Journal of Nursing Scholarship, 25*(4), 291–296.

Hancock, H., & Easen, P. (2006). The decision-making processes of nurses when extubating patients following cardiac surgery: An ethnographic study. *International Journal of Nursing Studies, 43*(6), 693–705.

Hoadley, T. (2009). Learning advanced cardiac life support: A comparison study of the effects of low and high fidelity simulation. *Nursing Education Perspectives, 30*, 91–95.

Houser, J. (2008). *Nursing research: Reading, using, and creating evidence.* Sudbury, MA: Jones and Bartlett.

Keele, R. (2009). Development of the exercise motivation questionnaire with Mexican-American adults. *Journal of Nursing Measurement, 17*, 183–194.

Lincoln, Y., & Guba, E. (1985). *Naturalistic inquiry.* Newbury Park, CA: Sage Publications.

McAuliffe, A. (2007). Nursing students' practice in providing oral hygiene for patients. *Nursing Standard, 21*, 35–39.

Reb, A. (2007). Transforming the death sentence: Elements of hope in women with advanced ovarian cancer. *Oncology Nursing Forum, 34*(6), E70–81.

Sandelowski, M. (1995). Focus on qualitative methods: Sample size in qualitative research. *Research in Nursing & Health, 18*, 179–183.

Sandelowski, M. (1986). The problem of rigor in qualitative research. *Advances in Nursing Science, 8*, 27–37.

Sengane, M. L., & Cur, D. (2009). The experience of black fathers concerning support for their wives/partners during labour. *Curationis, 32*(1), 67–73.

Siegel, J., & Korniewicz, D. (2007). Keeping patients safe: An interventional hand-hygiene study at an oncology center. *Clinical Journal of Oncology Nursing, 11*, 643–646.

Tanner, C., Benner, P., Chesla, C., & Gordon, D. (1993). The phenomenology of knowing the patient. *Journal of Nursing Scholarship, 25*, 273–280.

Tousman, S., Arnold, D., Helland, W., Roth, R., Heshelman, N., Castaneda, O., et al. (2007). Evaluation of a hand washing program for second graders. *The Journal of School Nursing, 23*, 342–348.

CHAPTER 4

Data Analysis

Once the data have been collected in a quantitative research design, statistical analyses are used to answer the research questions. To reiterate from Chapter 1, it is not necessary to comprehend all of the mathematical steps of the statistical procedures. What is more important, given the software and technology available to producers and consumers of research, is how to interpret the results in light of the research questions and the study design. Understanding both the descriptive and inferential statistics is important to accomplish this. The statistical information presented in this chapter is provided for the purpose of analyzing published research studies rather than performing statistical analyses yourself. To analyze the statistical analysis of a quantitative research study, you will need to be able to do the following:

1. Identify the statistical analyses performed.
2. Judge whether they were appropriate and matched the research design and questions/hypotheses/purpose of the study.
3. Judge whether the level of measurement matched the statistical test done.
4. Judge whether the interpretation of the statistical analyses made sense.
5. Evaluate not only the statistical significance of the findings but also the clinical significance of the findings.

These elements will be covered in the pages to follow in this chapter. It is impossible to cover every possible statistical test that you may see in published research. More importantly, it is unrealistic to expect you to memorize all of them; therefore, only the top 10 statistics published in nursing research as recommended by Zellner, Boerst, and Tabb (2007) will be covered in detail in this book.

Zellner et al. (2007) reviewed 462 quantitative research articles published in 13 nursing journals in 2000. A three-step process identified the nursing journals used in this study. First, the authors used the "Brandon/Hill Selected List of Print Nursing Books and Journals" by Hill and Stickell (2002). This list also included a comprehensive list of journals identified as key holdings for any library. The second step was to cross-reference these journals with the *Key and Electronic Nursing Journals: Characteristics and Database Coverage*, 2001 ed. (KENJ). This is a comprehensive guide of more than 200 national and international nursing journals (Allen, 2001). The third step included identifying which of these journals included an annual percentage of 40% or more of published research articles.

Authors of the reviewed studies consistently reported using similar statistical methods. **Table 4-1** presents the top 10 list of statistical methods used in published nursing research studies (Zellner et al., 2007). Although most researchers used these most common statistical procedures, there were some that used lesser-known statistical tests. Therefore, it is helpful to have on hand a comprehensive handbook of statistical methods as a reference tool when needed. A discussion of these 10 frequently used statistical methods will be presented based on the following categories of statistical tests: descriptive statistics (measures of central tendency and dispersion) and inferential statistics (parametric and nonparametric).

Table 4-1   Top 10 List of Statistical Methods Used in Nursing Research

1. Mean
2. Frequency distribution
3. Standard deviation
4. Range
5. Percentages, percentiles, quartiles
6. T-tests, independent and dependent
7. Analysis of Variance (ANOVA), all kinds
8. Correlation
9. Cronbach's alpha
10. Chi-Square

The top 10 methods represent approximately 80% of all statistical measures used in the 462 articles that were reviewed by Zellner, Boerst, & Tabb (2007).

DESCRIPTIVE STATISTICS

Descriptive statistics are important for summarizing and describing the study sample. Descriptive statistics include frequencies, measures of central tendency, and measures of variability. Before you can really understand even descriptive statistics, a beginning level of knowledge of frequency distributions and levels of measurement is important first.

Frequency Distributions

A frequency distribution reveals the lowest and highest scores and where most of the scores tend to cluster. Most statistical software programs such as SPSS (Statistical Package Social Sciences) can easily produce frequency data as histograms. See **Figure 4-1** for an example histogram. In this example, you can see that the age group with the most participants in this research study was the 18–20 year olds. Visual depictions of frequency information are a quick and easy way to get an idea of the demographics of the whole sample, in this case age. This histogram can also be called a distribution, which is defined as the

Figure 4-1   Sample histogram using age.

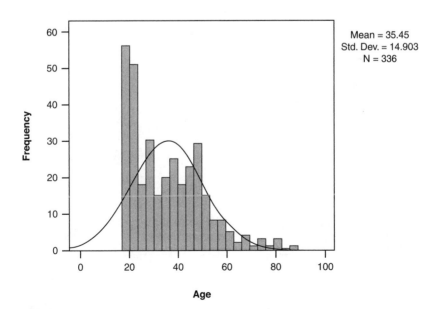

way that the variable of interest is clustered or spread across its continuum. It is the shape of the data when the data are graphed so that the levels of the variable are on the x-axis and the number of cases found at each data point is on the y-axis.

Symmetrical distributions, often called the bell curve, are shaped so that if divided into halves, the halves could be folded over one another and would fit almost exactly together. Skewed distributions have off-center peaks with longer tails in one direction. If the longer tail is on the right, it is called positively skewed; if the longer tail is on the left, it is called negatively skewed. See **Figure 4-2** for a symmetrical or normal distribution and **Figure 4-3** for examples of skewed or nonnormal distributions. An example of data that would appear as a skewed distribution would be the age of a group of Alzheimer's patients, since the majority would be older, thus pulling the hump to the right with a long tail toward the left and making it a negatively skewed distribution.

Levels of Measurement

There are four types of measurement scales: nominal, ordinal, interval, and ratio. As one moves up the levels (nominal to ratio), the level of precision of the measurement increases. Further, each level subsumes the characteristics of all of the levels below it and also adds a new quality.

Figure 4-2   Symmetrical or normal distribution.

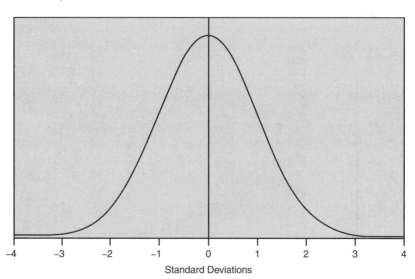

Standard Deviations

Retrieved April 20, 2010 from http://www.itl.nist.gov/div898/handbook/pmc/section5/pmc51.htm

Figure 4-3   Examples of skewed distributions.

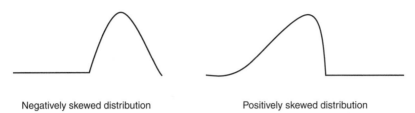

Negatively skewed distribution   Positively skewed distribution

Retrieved March 10, 2010 from http://www.kwiznet.com/p/takeQuiz.php?ChapterID=12045&
CurriculumID=42&Num=9.29

The least precise scale or level of data is the nominal scale. With a nominal scale, the numbers assigned to a variable have no quantitative meaning. This type of scale is used commonly with demographic information such as gender. For example, 1 can equal female and 2 can equal male or vice versa. The number does not mean anything other than a way to assign numbers to a variable. However, in the example just given with gender, 2 is not greater than 1. The number does not carry any qualities of greater than or less than or make any inferences about intervals between data points. However, once the numbers are assigned to males versus females, statistically a frequency distribution can be performed to demonstrate the mode—or which one (males or females) is the most representative in that sample.

The next level of data is the ordinal scale. Ordinal scales are used to rank data that are supposed to demonstrate greater than or less than. However, these scales do not provide information about the distance between the data points or between the highs and the lows. A commonly used ordinal scale is the visual analogue scale (VAS) for pain. See **Figure 4-4** for this scale.

An interval scale consists of all of the qualities of a nominal and ordinal scale plus it adds the quality of equal distance between data points or intervals. This characteristic allows the researcher to make conclusions regarding actual differences between measures rather than just saying that one measure is greater than another measure. Most standardized psychological tests used in nursing research studies are interval scales. Blood pressure and temperature are other examples. Even though there is some debate among researchers, most researchers agree that one of the most common summative rating scales, the Likert scale, is an interval scale. A Likert scale consists of several declarative statements that express an attitude or belief on a topic. Respondents typically are asked to indicate the degree of agreement or disagreement with each statement. The number of categories may range from four to seven. For

Figure 4-4   Sample visual analog scales for pain.

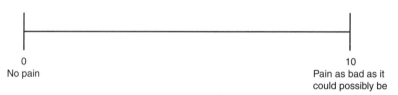

PAIN SCALE

No pain   Moderate pain   Worst pain

0   10
No pain   Pain as bad as it
                                                             could possibly be

From McCaffrey, M., & Pasero, C. (1999). *Pain: Clinical manual* (pp. 62–67). St. Louis, MO: Mosby, Inc.

example, the four category scale would include the following choices: strongly disagree, disagree, agree, and strongly agree. Respondents are asked to select only one category that best reflects their feelings regarding each statement. Each category is assigned a numerical value so that the data can be analyzed. Commonly, in the 1–4 category scale described here, strongly disagree would equal 1, disagree would equal 2, agree would equal 3, and strongly agree would equal 4. Scores for each item would be summed across the total scale or by subscale depending on the design of the instrument. Examples of items that could be included on a Likert scale include: "I exercise because it is important to my health" or "I exercise because my partner wants me to."

A ratio scale subsumes all of the qualities of the other measurement scales (naming, ranking, equal intervals) plus it adds the quality of an absolute zero point. It is considered the most precise measurement scale. Examples of ratio scales include time, length, and weight. It is important to note that ratio scales are hard to come by because they do require the quality of an absolute zero point or absence of the quality. Many ratio scales are found in biologic measures rather than psychosocial measures.

The more precise the measurement scale, the more precise the data collected using that scale. Further, the more precise the data are, the more amenable the data are to the most powerful and sophisticated statistical analyses. Stronger statistical tests can be done if there is at least interval or ratio data.

Measures of Central Tendency

Measures of central tendency include the mean, median, and mode. The mean or "average" is the most commonly used measure of central tendency. The mean is calculated by adding all of the scores together and then dividing by the number of scores being summed. The median is the midpoint or middle score of the distribution and divides the scores into two halves. It is calculated by arranging the scores in increasing order and finding the score where half of the scores are above it and half are below it. The mode is the most frequent score in a set of data. For example if you had a set of scores that included 5, 5, 3, 4, 5, the mode would be 5 since it is the most frequently occurring score.

The mode is the only useful measure of central tendency when a variable is measured on a nominal scale. A typical example, provided by McHugh (2003), is a pediatric nurse practitioner keeping record of the final diagnosis of the 100 children who came in during one of the winter months with the following symptoms: clear runny nose, fever, generalized aching of the muscles of the body, and either lethargy or irritability. The distribution might look like the one in **Figure 4-5**. In this distribution 1 represents seasonal flu, 2 is swine flu, 3 is

Figure 4-5   Histogram demonstrating use of mode with childhood diagnoses.

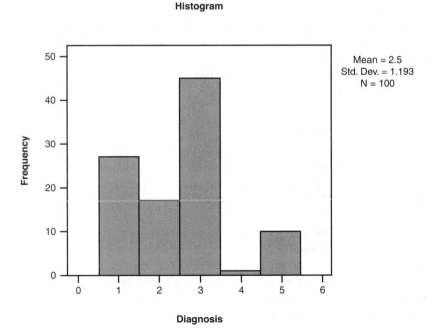

the common cold, 4 is pneumonia, and 5 is ear infection. From this distribution, it can be seen that the most common diagnosis was a cold.

For ordinal data, the median is the best indicator of central tendency. One of the advantages of the median is its insensitivity to extreme scores. This can work as an advantage particularly with skewed or nonnormal distributions. For example, a set of knowledge scores on a diabetes test was 80, 85, 90, 95, and 100. The median score is 90. If we change one of these scores to reflect an extreme score compared to the others, we might have 20, 85, 90, 95, and 100. The median is still 90 even with the extreme score of 20. Thus, in skewed distributions with extreme scores, the median is the appropriate measure of central tendency to use.

The mean is a very powerful measure of central tendency. Of all the measures of central tendency, the mean is viewed as the most reliable and stable. It incorporates the exact score from every subject into its estimate of central tendency. However, when some scores are extreme, as depicted in the example above, the mean is extremely sensitive to these extreme scores and can become distorted. It was demonstrated by changing the 80 to a score of 20 that the median did not change in the data set. However, if you calculate the mean on the first data set, it is 90. If you only change one score as was done in the second data set with an extreme score, the mean now changes to a score of 78. This is why the mean is not the appropriate measure of central tendency to use with skewed distributions, but it can be very powerful with normal distributions where extreme scores cannot unduly influence it.

Nominal and ordinal data are often labeled *categorical* because there are a limited discrete number of data points within the data. Nominal measures use the mode as the appropriate measure of central tendency in statistical tests. Ordinal measures typically use the median. Interval and ratio measures/data require the mean and a normal distribution.

Measures of Variability

Variability refers to how the scores are dispersed throughout the entire range of the variable within the distribution. If the scores in a data set are similar, there is very little variability. A measure of central tendency without a corresponding measure of variability provides limited information about the distribution (Wilson, 1993). Measures of central tendency provide information about ways subjects are grouped together, whereas measures of variability give information about how the scores are spread out or separated.

The two most common measures of variability are the range and the standard deviation. The range is the least precise measure of variability. It is calculated by subtracting the lowest score from the highest score in the distribution. As you can see, this measure is easy to calculate but a relatively crude measure since one extreme score can influence it. For example, you can have two sets of data that are the same except for one score. If one score is a lot higher than the scores in the other data set, the range will be very different. The range lets the researcher know how widely the subjects actually scored across the possible range of values. It does not tell the researcher if cases were evenly spread across the possible values or if there were clumps of scores and scores not represented by the dataset. The variance and the standard deviation provide better descriptions of average variability in the dataset.

If each of the scores in the dataset is subtracted from the mean, we would have an idea of how much each of the scores deviated from the mean. However, if we try to sum those scores to get an average deviation, we find that it will not work since the sum of these scores always equals zero. So, it is necessary to square each of these deviations. The sum of the squared deviations can be divided by the sample size or number of data points to obtain an average deviation, which is called variance. Variance by itself is rather limited since it is now in squared units and is not the original measure. Thus, the best option is to the take the square root of the variance to eliminate this problem with the result being the standard deviation. In the example presented in **Table 4-2**, the sum of squares is 3475. The variance is calculated by dividing the sum of squares by the mean (3475/52.5 = 66.19).

The standard deviation, another measure of variability, examines how scores vary or are dispersed about the mean. It is considered a reliable estimate of the amount a "typical" score varies from the mean. The standard deviation is calculated by taking the square root of the variance. In the example provided in Table 4-2, the standard deviation equals 8.14.

A small standard deviation means that most of the scores cluster tightly around the mean. Approximately 68% of the participants lie between one standard deviation above and below the mean of any distribution. Ninety-five percent of scores will fall within two standard deviations above and below the

Table 4-2   Obtaining Variance and Standard Deviation of a Set of Numbers

Participant's Score	Mean	Score minus mean	(Score minus mean)^2
20	52.5	−32.5	1056.25
50	52.5	−2.5	6.25
40	52.5	−12.5	156.25
100	52.5	47.5	2256.25
Total: 210	Mean: 210/4 = 52.5		Total: 3475

mean. The majority (99%) of participants will fall within three standard deviations above and below the mean (Figure 4-2). Two sets of scores can have the same mean but have very different standard deviations. For example, two groups of subjects take the same depression questionnaire. One group has chronic pain, and the other group does not. It is found the mean scores are the same on the depression scores, but the standard deviations are very different. The chronic pain group has a standard deviation of 2 whereas the group without pain has a standard deviation of 9. Since the chronic pain group is more similar than the other group on the variable measured by the depression score, the standard deviation was much less.

Percentage distributions indicate the percentage of the sample whose scores fall into a specific group along with the number of scores in that group. Percentage distributions can be particularly useful for comparing the present data with findings from other studies with different sample sizes (Burns & Grove, 2003).

It can be useful at times to know where a particular participant's score falls relative to the entire distribution. A percentile is the best statistic for this purpose and is commonly used in nursing research studies. A percentile orders all of the scores from highest to lowest and calculates the percentage of scores that fall below each of the individual scores. A quartile is the entire percentile chart divided into four equal sections. Scores from the 75th to 99th percentile form the top quartile. The 50th to the 74th percentile form the second highest quartile. Scores from the 26th to the 49th percentile form the third quartile, and scores from the 1st to the 25th percentile form the lowest quartile (McHugh, 2003).

INFERENTIAL STATISTICS

Descriptive statistics are commonly insufficient to answer the study's research questions. Inferential statistics are statistical procedures used to answer research questions within a study with the goal of inferring these findings back to the target population from which the sample was taken. Inferential statistics are a test on one of the measures of central tendency; mean, median, or mode. There are two main categories of inferential statistics; parametric and nonparametric statistical tests.

Parametric Statistical Tests

To perform the stronger and more powerful parametric tests, several requirements have to be met. Requirements include a normal distribution of scores, minimum of interval level data, and an estimation of at least one parameter (a characteristic of a population such as mean age of the subjects in a study).

Some of the more commonly used parametric statistical tests include T-tests, analysis of variance (ANOVA), correlations, multiple regression, and multivariate analysis of variance (MANOVA).

Parametric tests are tests on mean differences, which is why there must be a minimum of interval level data. Sometimes the researcher is interested in testing differences between different groups of subjects (between subjects design) on the dependent or outcome measure. This type of design uses independent samples in that the groups of subjects contain different people. In the hand washing example from Chapter 1, the research questions included:

Does a multifaceted interventional hand-hygiene program positively affect healthcare workers' compliance with hand washing guidelines in an ICU?

Does a multifaceted interventional hand-hygiene program positively affect healthcare workers' attitudes, beliefs, and knowledge about hand washing guidelines?

To review, in the first research question, the hand-hygiene program is the treatment or independent variable and rate of hand washing compliance by healthcare workers is the dependent variable. In the second question, the independent variable is the same, but the dependent variables are workers' attitudes, beliefs, and knowledge about hand washing guidelines. The researcher may be interested in testing whether nurses did better than physicians on hand washing compliance after the hand washing intervention. An independent samples T-test or analysis of variance (ANOVA) would be the statistical test of choice. When you have only two groups, these two tests yield the same results. If you have three or more groups, the ANOVA should be used since the T-test is only for two groups. However, the research question in the same example is primarily asking if the hand-hygiene intervention increased hand washing compliance. Since the subjects are the same, just measure before and after the hand washing intervention, it is called a within-subjects design. For this design, a paired samples T-test would be the statistical test of choice.

If the research question is not trying to test for differences but to examine relationships between variables, a correlation coefficient is performed. A correlation addresses the extent that two variables are related to each other in a linear fashion. For example, "To what extent is a diet high in fat related to obesity?" Correlation analyses provide information about both the direction and the strength of relationship between variables. Correlation coefficients can vary from a positive 1 to a negative 1. A correlation of 0 indicates no relationship, whereas correlations closer to positive or negative 1 indicate strong relationships. Correlations of positive or negative 1 indicate a perfect correlation. The visual presentation of the relationship between two variables is called a scatter plot. Each point represents the point of each participant's values or scores on a variable on the x- and y-axes. These scatter plots indicate both the direction and strength of the relationship between variables. The more the dots line up in a straight line at a 45° angle to the axes, the higher the correlation (see **Figure 4-6** for sample scatter plots). A positive or direct relationship indicates that as one variable increases, the other one does also. In the sample question above, if there were a positive relationship, the interpretation would

Figure 4-6 Sample scatter plots.

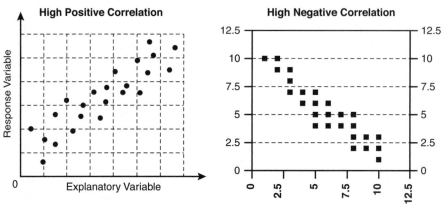

Indicates a very strong positive relationship between variables

Indicates a very strong negative relationship between variables

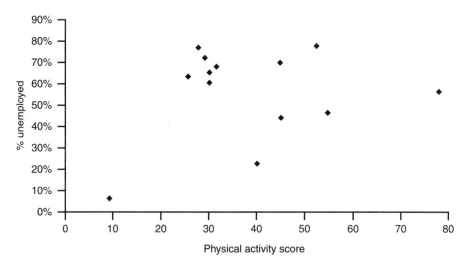

Indicates a very weak if any relationship between the variables

Retrieved March 10, 2010 from http://www.netmba.com/images/statistics/plot/scatter/scatterplot.gif.

be "as a diet high in fat increases, so does the risk of obesity." A negative or indirect relationship would indicate that as the value of one variable increases, the other one decreases. In the same example, this would be interpreted "as a diet high in fat increases, the risk of obesity decreases." One of the most common types of correlation coefficients is the Pearson's r. For example, the following research question could be asked: "What is the relationship between smoking and incidence of lung cancer?" A correlation coefficient of 0.7 would indicate a strong positive relation. That is, as smoking increases, so does the incidence of lung cancer. If the following research question: "What is the relationship between physical activity and depression?" resulted in a correlation coefficient of -0.6, it would be interpreted as a strong negative correlation. That is, as levels of physical activity increase, depression scores would decrease.

In multiple regression, more than one independent variable is used to predict the dependent variable. For example, if the researcher is interested in determining what best predicts exercise motivation, they may collect data on independent variables such as social support, weight, past experience with exercise, age, and current health status. Statistically, the regression analysis indicates the amount of variance in the data explained by the independent variables in the analysis. Each of the independent variables can be put into the equation in a stepwise fashion (i.e., social support, then weight, etc.) to evaluate the impact of each variable separately and then in conjunction with the other variables in the equation.

Nonparametric Statistical Tests

If any of these requirements were not met, then the appropriate category of statistical tests would be the nonparametric, since there are no strict requirements regarding shape of distribution. Called "distribution-free" tests, nonparametric statistical tests are the category of choice when there is a skewed or nonnormal distribution. Commonly used nonparametric tests include chi-square, Mann-Whitney U, Wilcoxon signed-rank test, logistic regression, and Spearman's rho.

The chi-square (χ^2) is one of the most frequently used nonparametric statistics reported in nursing research. This test is appropriate when you have nominal data, and you are interested in whether the data falls within two or more categories within an expected pattern. Examples of common nominal data in nursing research include demographic information such as gender, marital status, health status, and ethnicity.

The Mann-Whitney U is the nonparametric form of the independent samples T-test looks, but the Mann-Whitney is used for ordinal data. The Wilcoxon signed-rank test is the nonparametric form of the paired samples T-test, and only ordinal data can be obtained. Logistic regression is the nonparametric form of multiple regression where only ordinal level data can be obtained. Lastly, Spearman's rho is the nonparametric version of a Pearson's r when interval or ratio data cannot be obtained but the researcher is interested in testing relationships between independent and dependent variables.

CHOOSING THE APPROPRIATE STATISTICAL TEST

Choice of statistics depends upon several considerations. Of course, as already discussed, the research question should drive the design, which then directs the rest of the study. For example, if the research question is, "What is the impact of hourly rounding on adverse events on patients in a hospital?" it requires collecting data on these adverse events before and after the implementation of hourly rounding. Statistically, a test that examines differences would be selected, such as a T-test rather than a test that examines relationships (i.e., correlation coefficient). Another very important consideration is the measurement scale or level of data that the data collection instrument(s) produced. As already discussed, nominal and ordinal data are considered categorical data, and interval and ratio data are considered continuous data. Nonparametric tests are appropriate for categorical data especially if the distribution is skewed. Parametric tests are appropriate for continuous data if the distribution is normal. See **Table 4-3** for a guide in matching design with level of data and examples of appropriate statistical tests. Carlson, Protsman, and Tomaka (2005) provide more guides in their graphic organizers. **Figure 4-7** presents

---

Table 4-3   Matching Research Design to Major Components of the Research Process

Nonexperimental quantitative designs	Experimental-level quantitative designs
Level 1 or Level 2 inquiry research question(s):	Level 3 or Level 4 inquiry research question(s):
• Sampling usually nonprobability sampling such as convenience or purposive sampling	• Sampling usually probability sampling (randomized in some way either through initial selection or random assignment into treatment groups)
• Level of data mainly categorical (nominal/ordinal)	• Need power analysis to determine sample size
• Statistical analysis mainly descriptive (e.g., frequencies, percentages, nonparametric tests on the median)	• Level of data mainly interval and ratio but may have some nominal and ordinal data
	• Statistical analysis mainly parametric tests such as ANOVA, T-test, regression, Pearson's correlations

Table 4-3   **Matching Research Design to Major Components of the Research Process** *(continued)*

Nonexperimental quantitative designs	Experimental-level quantitative designs
Specific examples:	**Specific examples:**
Descriptive level design	**Quasi-experimental design**
Two groups	Two groups
Level 1 inquiry	Level 3 inquiry
Convenience sample	Nonprobability sampling such as convenience sampling
Nominal and ordinal data	Interval or ratio data
Descriptive statistics such as percentages to describe the sample and chi-square performed to determine differences between the two groups	There is usually a treatment
	Parametric tests to test the mean difference between the two groups such as T-tests
	If more than two groups, then you would need to do ANOVA
Correlation level design	**Experimental designs**
Two groups	Two or more groups
Level 2 inquiry	Level 4 inquiry
Convenience sample	Random sampling
Ordinal or interval level data	Interval or ratio data
Nonparametric correlation such as Wilcoxon or McNemars if ordinal level data	There is usually a treatment
Parametric correlation such as Pearson's correlation if interval level data	Parametric tests to test mean differences. If only two groups, then tests such as T-test would be appropriate. If more than two groups, then tests such as ANOVA and regression would be appropriate. Multivariate tests would also be appropriate, such as MANOVA or multiple regression.

an algorithm for nominal and ordinal data. **Figures 4-8** and **4-9** are algorithms for interval and ratio data depending on how many independent variables are involved. If we take the example on hourly rounding, the research question is, "What is the impact of hourly rounding on adverse events on patients in a hospital?" Data would be collected on mean number of adverse events before and after the implementation of hourly rounding. The independent variable is hourly rounding and mean number of adverse events is the dependent variable. The groups are dependent since it is the same subjects being compared before and after implementation of the hourly rounding. There are two groups, one

Figure 4-7   Graphic organizer for nominal and ordinal data.

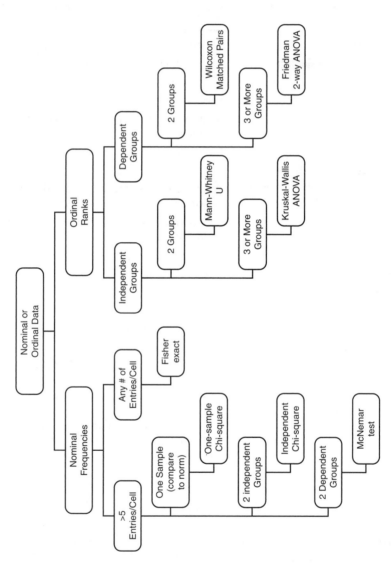

From Carlson, M., Protsman, L., & Tomaka, J. (2005). Graphic organizers can facilitate selection of statistical tests, part 1: Analysis of group differences. *Journal of Physical Therapy Education, 19,* 57–65.

Figure 4-8   Graphic organizer for interval/ratio data with one independent variable.

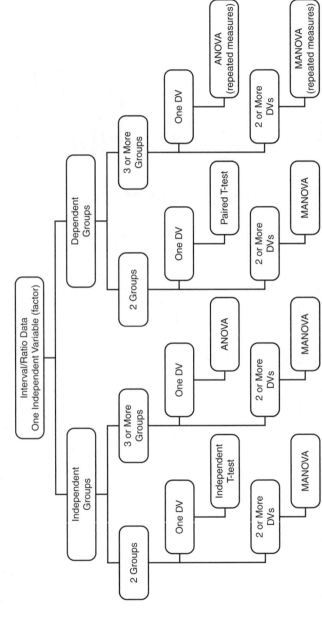

From Carlson, M., Protsman, L., & Tomaka, J. (2005). Graphic organizers can facilitate selection of statistical tests, part 1: Analysis of group differences. *Journal of Physical Therapy Education, 19,* 57–65.

Figure 4-9   Graphic organizer for interval/ratio data with two or more independent variables.

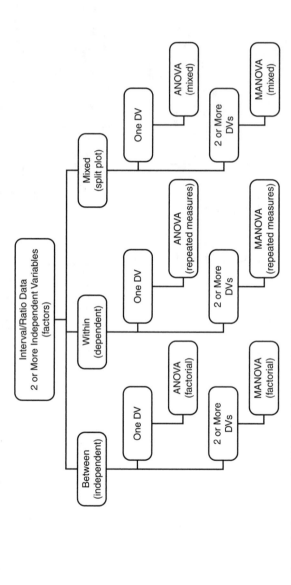

From Carlson, M., Protsman, L., & Tomaka, J. (2005). Graphic organizers can facilitate selection of statistical tests, part 1: Analysis of group differences. *Journal of Physical Therapy Education, 19,* 57–65.

independent and one dependent variable. Using the algorithm provided in Figure 4-8 for interval/ratio data with one independent variable, the appropriate statistical test is the paired T-test.

INTERPRETING STATISTICAL TESTS

Interpreting the *p* value

A *p* value is a probability that determines whether a difference between two or more interventions is statistically significant enough to change the current standard of care. The researcher sets the level of significance of a study before the study begins. The normally acceptable level of significance is 0.05. This can be interpreted as "the probability that significant differences will be found between groups on the treatment/intervention by chance alone is 5 out of 100 times." This is the probability of committing a type I error discussed in Chapter 2. If the treatment could cause adverse effects or even death, the level of significance might be set even smaller by the researcher, such as 0.01. This would be interpreted as "the probability that significant differences will be found between groups on the treatment/intervention by chance alone is only 1 out of 100 times." However, if we make the significance level too small and rigid, we may decrease our chances of making a type I error but increase our chances of making a type II error. In other words, as you make one more rigid/smaller, you make the other more relaxed/larger. So, as a researcher, a decision has to be made as to how critical it is to not make a type I error but still not jeopardize committing a type II if possible. To reiterate, the acceptable norm is 0.05 for the predetermined significance level but may be made more stringent if the treatment can cause undue harm or even death if a type I error is made (saying that the experimental treatment is effective when in reality it is not).

Interpretation of Results

Interpretation of results from quasi-experimental and experimental designs includes five possible results:

1. Significant findings as predicted by the researcher
2. Nonsignificant findings
3. Mixed results
4. Unexpected results
5. Significant results that are opposite those predicted by the researcher

Significant results confirm those predicted initially by the researcher. Nonsignificant results, often called "negative results" are not confirming the predicted results. Many times, particularly in nursing research, this is not due to lack of significant or effective interventions but due to too small of a sample size or questionable validity and reliability of the data gathering instruments. Mixed results are very common in nursing research and may be related to flaws in methodology or application of theory. Unexpected results are results found between variables that were not initially hypothesized. Significant results opposite of those predicted indicate possible flaws in thinking by both the researcher and the theory being tested.

Statistical Significance Versus Clinical Significance

Consumers of research have the difficult task of making sense out of a study's findings, including discerning between statistical significance and clinical significance. Many times a study will report statistically significant findings but cannot make a good argument about how relevant they are to clinical practice. Studies that have huge sample sizes and multiple statistical tests at multiple data points increase their chances of getting statistical significance, but the differences between groups are so small that it does not make sense clinically. Oliver and Mahon (2005) provide an example where this is the case. The study was comparing two groups of patients newly diagnosed with breast cancer. The hypothesis of the study was whether a support group would have a positive effect on the overall well-being of patients in the experimental group over the course of treatment. Demographic data such as age, education, health status, race, religion, and living arrangements were collected. Scores on quality of life and functional measures were compared at several points. Results of a T-test revealed that the mean age between the control and experimental groups was statistically significant, with more older women in the control group. However, this does not necessarily imply that a clinical difference exists. The consumer must discern whether having more older subjects in one group could bias or confound the study's interpretation of findings. A difference might exist because the older women most likely would be postmenopausal or menopausal, whereas the younger subjects may or may not be. Therefore, issues of menopause could confound the results. Keele-Smith and Price-Daniel (2001) conducted a study on the effects of crossing legs on blood pressure with older adults and found that blood pressure was statistically significantly higher when legs were crossed versus uncrossed. Systolic pressure changed by 5.9 mm Hg, and the diastolic pressure changed by 2.97. Even though this was a small change, it was statistically significant. The authors argued that this change, however small, was clinically relevant, particularly in the older adult population used in this study.

THE BIG "SO WHAT?"

- Interpretation of a study's findings and its relation to practice is more important than knowing all of the mathematical formulas involved in statistical analyses.

- To analyze the statistical analysis of a quantitative study, you need to be able to identify the analyses performed, ensure a match between design and the analyses and level of measurement of data collected, and judge whether the interpretation and application of findings was done appropriately.
- There are 10 top statistics published in nursing research studies.
- There are four levels of measurement, with each subsequent level subsuming the qualities of the earlier levels.
- The four levels of measurement include, from lowest to highest level: nominal, ordinal, interval, and ratio.
- Measures of central tendency include the mode, median, and mean.
- The two most common measures of variability are the range and the standard deviation.
- Descriptive statistics are important for summarizing and describing the sample.
- Normal distributions where interval data can be assumed are critical for calculating means and performing the stronger parametric statistical tests.
- Some of the more common parametric statistical tests include the T-test, ANOVA, correlation, and multiple regression.
- If a skewed or nonnormal distribution is present, then nominal and ordinal data may be assumed and only the nonparametric statistical tests can be correctly performed.
- Some of the most common nonparametric statistical tests are the chi-square, Mann-Whitney U, Wilcoxon signed-rank, logistic regression, and Spearman's rho.
- Algorithms can be used to assist with proper choice of statistical test.
- A p value is a probability that determines whether a difference between two or more interventions is statistically significant enough to change the current standard of care.
- Level of significance is the way to control for type I errors.
- A researcher does not want to commit either a type I or type II error.
- If you decrease your chances of making a type I error, you increase your chance of making a type II error.
- You can have statistical significance without clinical significance.

REFERENCES

Allen, M. (2007). *Key and electronic nursing journals: Characteristics and database coverage.* Retrieved from http://www.utexas.edu/nursing/norr/docs/keyjournals07.pdf

Burns, N., & Grove, S. (2003). *Understanding nursing research* (3rd ed.). Philadelphia, PA: Saunders.

Carlson, M., Protsman, L., & Tomaka, J. (2005). Graphic organizers can facilitate selection of statistical tests, part 1: Analysis of group differences. *Journal of Physical Therapy Education, 19*, 57–65.

Hill, D., & Stickell, H. (2002). Brandon/Hill selected list of print nursing books and journals. *Nursing Outlook, 50*, 100–113.

Keele-Smith, R., & Price-Daniel, C. (2001). Effects of crossing legs on blood pressure measurement. *Clinical Nursing Research, 10*, 202–213.

McCaffrey, M., & Pasero, C. (1999). *Pain: Clinical manual* (pp. 62–67). St. Louis, MO: Mosby.

McHugh, M. (2003). Descriptive statistics, part II: most commonly used descriptive statistics. *Journal for Specialists in Pediatric Nursing, 8*, 111–116.

Oliver, D., & Mahon, S. (2005). Reading a research article, part II: Parametric and nonparametric statistics. *Clinical Journal of Oncology Nursing, 9*, 238–240.

Wilson, H. S. (1993). *Introducing nursing research* (2nd ed.). Redwood City, CA: Addison-Wesley.

Zellner, K., Boerst, C., & Tabb, W. (2007). Statistics used in current nursing research. *Journal of Nursing Education, 46*, 55–59.

CHAPTER 5

Implementing Evidence-Based Nursing Practice: An Overview

GETTING STARTED

To start, let us review the definition and description of evidence-based nursing practice presented in Chapter 1. Evidence-based practice (EBP) definitions are varied, but all include evidence from three broad areas: empirical studies, other forms of published evidence (e.g., review articles, clinical pathways, protocols), available clinical expertise and resources, and patient preferences/nuisances. Melnyk and Fineout-Overholt (2005) define EBP as a problem-solving approach using current best evidence to answer a clinical question incorporating one's own clinical expertise and patient values and preferences. As I presented in Chapter 1, I would argue that a better term to differentiate the uniqueness of nursing practice from other disciplines would be evidence-based nursing practice (EBNP) and will refer to it as EBNP from this point on.

Evidence-Based Nursing Practice Models

Several models have contributed conceptually to the implementation of evidence-based nursing practice. The Stetler model (Stetler, 2001), the Iowa model (Titler et al., 2001), the John Hopkins Evidence-Based Practice Model (Newhouse, et al., 2007), the ACE Star Model (Stevens, 2004), the Caledonian Development Model (Tolson, Booth, & Lowndes, 2008), and the Evidence-Based Practice Model for Staff Nurses (Reavy & Tavernier, 2008). Three of the most common models used today are discussed next.

The Stetler model, first developed in 1976 and refined in 1994, went through an update in 2001. Five phases are included in the process of performing EBNP (Stetler, 2001):

1. Preparation—This phase includes the identification of the problem/issue and validation of the problem with evidence.

2. Validation—Critique and synthesis of the evidence (empirical and non-empirical evidence, systematic reviews, etc.). Rate the level and quality of each item of evidence using a "table of evidence." Eliminate noncredible sources. Process ends here if there is no evidence or it is clearly insufficient.
3. Comparative evaluation/Decision making—Synthesize the cumulative findings. Make a decision about what can be used. At this point, there is an option to conduct own research if findings cannot be used.
4. Translation/Application—Decide on what level of application (individual, group, organization). Develop proposal for practice change. Create strategies for formal dissemination and planned change. Consider a pilot project.
5. Evaluation—Evaluation can be formal or informal. Consider costs. Include both formative and summative evaluations of outcomes.

The Iowa model starts with a trigger/problem. These triggers may be knowledge focused or problem focused. If the problem is a priority for the organization, then a team is formed. The team is composed of key stakeholders, clinicians, staff nurses, and other champions of evidence-based practice. The next step is synthesizing the evidence. A pilot of the practice change occurs if there is sufficient evidence to support the change. Evaluation of outcomes and dissemination of findings would follow. The Iowa model is depicted in **Figure 5-1**.

Hermes et al. (2009) used the Iowa model to develop an evidence-based imminent suicide risk instrument. The trigger for the project began with the decision-making process for placing patients on suicide watch. Nurses questioned whether the current protocol was accurate in identifying patients at risk. The second step was determining if the topic was a priority for the organization. All members of the unit-based council believed it was important to examine the appropriateness of the current tool. The third step was to form a team, which included two staff nurses from the unit-based council to lead the team, two clinical nurses to complete the project, and the hospital's nursing research facilitator who served as advisor to the project. The fourth step involves assembling and analyzing the research. This process included 11 studies that addressed assessment of suicide risk in an inpatient setting. A grading schema used to grade the quality of evidence included the following system:

- A—evidence from well-designed meta-analysis or integrated literature reviews
- B—evidence from well-designed controlled trials, both randomized and nonrandomized
- C—evidence from observational studies, such as descriptive and correlational
- D—evidence from expert opinion or multiple case reports

Figure 5-1 The Iowa Model of Evidence-Based Practice to Promote Quality Care.

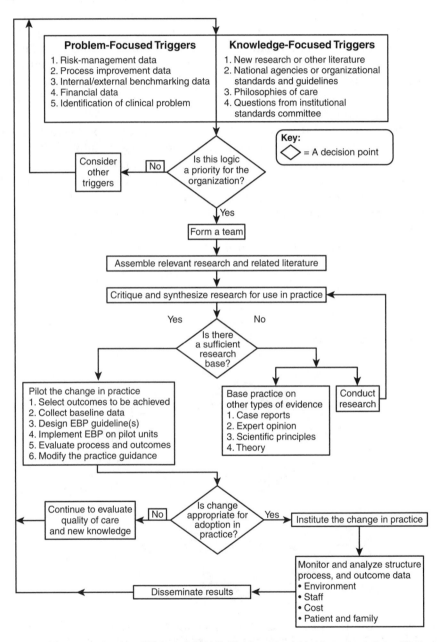

Reprinted with permission from Titler et al. (2001). The Iowa model evidence-based practice to promote quality care. *Critical Care Nursing Clinics of North America, 13*(4), 497–509. University of Iowa Hospitals and Clinics.

In the sample study, most evidence was rated C or D. A critical analysis of the evidence is part of the fourth step. The fifth step is determining if there is enough evidence to pilot the practice change. The team decided that there was sufficient evidence to move forward as a unit-based quality improvement initiative. The hospital librarian assisted with literature searches to find an instrument that would contain questions about suicide ideation but also assess for signs and symptoms of anxiety and agitation. The Behavioral Activity Rating Scale is helpful in assessing agitation in this patient population. Items from the Hamilton Anxiety Scale, used in a previous study on this unit, were added to the Behavioral Activity Rating Scale. A pilot test of this instrument followed. The sixth step is implementing the practice change into practice. This step included approval from the forms committee at the hospital and intensive in-service education for all staff nurses involved. To evaluate outcomes 6 weeks after the initial implementation, a representative of the unit-based council questioned staff nurses about their satisfaction with the new instrument.

The ACE (Academic Center for Evidence-Based Practice) Star Model is another frequently used evidence-based practice model. Visually depicted (**Figure 5-2**), it presents a framework for understanding the relationships between

Figure 5-2 The ACE Star Model.

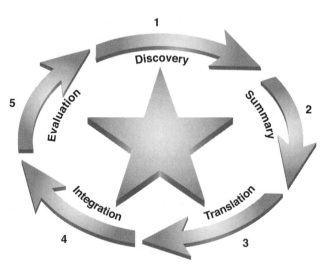

Reprinted with permission from Stevens, K. R. (2004). ACE Star Model of EPB: Knowledge Transformation. The University of Texas Health Science Center at San Antonio: Academic Center for Evidence-Based Practice.

various stages of knowledge transformation. Knowledge transformation is defined as the "conversion of research findings from primary research results, through a series of stages and forms, to impact on health outcomes by way of evidence-based care (Stevens, 2004)." It provides a framework for systematically putting evidence-based practice processes into action. Each point of the star represents a stage of knowledge transformation:

1. Knowledge discovery—new knowledge discovered through traditional empirical research including both quantitative and qualitative studies
2. Evidence summary—synthesizing across the research over a particular issue or problem; includes findings from systematic reviews and meta-analyses
3. Translation into practice recommendations—summarized research evidence is combined with other sources of evidence such as clinical expertise; then this holistic evidence is translated for the specific population and setting
4. Integration into practice—implementing the practice change through formal and informal methods; taking into account individual and organizational factors that affect adoption and integration into the system
5. Evaluation—includes the evaluation of the practice change on patient health outcomes and provider and client satisfaction

With the exception of the ACE Star Model, other models described in this discussion offer a sequential, step-wise approach to moving evidence into practice. By contrast, the ACE Star Model explains the very nature of the knowledge necessary to transform practice. As knowledge is translated into the next stage, it becomes increasingly useful and useable at the bedside and in direct patient care. Understanding the concepts in the ACE Star Model is fundamental to moving knowledge into clinical decision making (K. R. Stevens, personal communication, April 20, 2010).

Common threads woven across the majority of these evidence-based practice models include identification of the clinical problem through data gathering techniques, synthesizing the evidence, translating the evidence into a practice change, and implementation and evaluation of the practice change. Involvement of key stakeholders such as staff nurses plays an important role in these models. I would like to make the argument that having multiple models to choose from can make it difficult for the staff nurse. To compound the problem, there is lack of uniformity of terminology across the models. Complex terms, unique to each model, make it difficult to understand the process.

Even though the sample models of evidence-based practice described here provide needed guidelines for success, there are still challenges noted in the literature. It is still not clear what evidence should be used in the evidence-based nursing practice process. Historically, quantitative empirical research studies, particularly randomized controlled trials, were held as the highest level of evidence. Current literature suggests using a broader evidence base, which includes not only empirical quantitative studies but also qualitative research studies, clinical experience, patient experience, and information from the local context/organizational culture (Rycroft-Malone et al., 2004).

The evidence-based practice model that most mirrors this author's proposed guidelines for doing evidence-based nursing practice is the Evidence-Based Practice Model for Staff Nurses (Reavey & Tavernier, 2008). In this model, the authors integrated conceptual underpinnings from the Iowa model, the Stetler model and Rosswurm and Larrabee's (1999) model. The Iowa and Stetler models were discussed in some detail in earlier paragraphs. The Rosswurm and Larrabee model's primary focus is the application of change theory in implementing evidence-based practice. The uniqueness of the Evidence-Based Practice Model for Staff Nurses is its focus on the involvement of the staff nurse throughout the process. Recognition of the expertise that the staff nurse can bring to the table is a highlight of this model. Another important component of this model is the emphasis on communication throughout the process of evidence-based nursing practice.

The process for using the Evidence-Based Practice Model for Staff Nurses mirrors the nursing process with an assessment, diagnoses (identification of the problem), planning, implementation, and evaluation components. With the addition of analysis and synthesis of evidence, and integration and maintenance of practice change, the model is complete. Active input from patients, staff nurses, and nurse researchers is a key component of its successful implementation. Communication between the staff nurses, patients, and nurse researchers is pivotal to successful implementation of this model.

Reavey and Tavernier (2008) share an example of how their model was implemented, starting with a team formation of staff nurses, unit nurse manager, clinical nurse specialist, nurse researcher, and infection control nurse. The clinical problem selected was determining the best practice for frequency of central line dressing changes in severely neutropenic patients. The current policy required daily dressing changes. However, daily dressing changes resulted in skin breakdown that increased the potential for infection. Further, the clients were dissatisfied with the frequency due to the discomfort the skin breakdown caused. The next task for the team included a literature search of available evidence. The nurse researcher and the clinical nurse specialist took the lead in this step due to the heavy workloads, inadequate time, and lack of knowledge problems voiced by the staff nurses. Based on the evidence, the team proposed that central line dressings be changed every 7 days or as needed, except for gauze dressings, which need to be changed every 2 days. Projected outcomes were reduced costs due to fewer supplies needed and less nursing time required, along with decreased infections and skin breakdown. Implementation, done by the team, included education for all of the staff nurses, conducting a pilot study, and measuring outcomes. During the 6 months following implementation of the practice change, the bloodstream infection rate remained below the benchmark of 4 per 1,000 line days (Reavy & Tavernier, 2008).

I would like to take the argument related to evidence-based practice models I started a short while back even further at this point. If the nursing profession supports evidence-based nursing practice and expects all professional nurses (even at the bedside) to practice it, then I would suggest that the process be made as user-friendly as possible. I propose the following 10 steps that provide a systematic approach to collecting and synthesizing all of the needed forms of evidence and for creating EBNP changes to improve the quality of patient care:

1. Identifying the practice problem/issue
2. Collecting and appraising the empirical evidence
3. Collecting and appraising the nonempirical evidence
4. Summarizing across all of the evidence
5. Integrating the evidence with clinical expertise, client preferences, and values in making a proposed practice change or decision
6. Developing the proposed practice change in detail
7. Considering feasibility and organizational issues
8. Evaluating the practice change
9. Marketing the practice change
10. Strategies for successful implementation and sustainability of practice change

Detail related to each step is presented in **Table 5-1**. It is important to note at this point that evidence-based nursing practice cannot be done in isolation. Involvement from key stakeholders or champions, including representation from the target population, is mandatory for successful implementation. To prevent evidence-based nursing practice from being "cookbook" nursing, the nurse must decide how to incorporate patient preferences/values into the practice change for any particular patient (DiCenso, Cullum, & Ciliska, 1998). This might include making the decision that the practice change needs adapting to that particular patient. Further, these authors suggest that the incorporation of clinical expertise be balanced with the risks and benefits of treatment options for each patient. Further, there is a need to take into account the patient's unique circumstances such as comorbid conditions and preferences (DiCenso, Cullum, & Ciliska, 1998). Now, let us take each of these steps and discuss in more detail.

Table 5-1   Outline of the 10 Steps for Creating EBP Changes

---

1. Identifying the practice problem/issue
2. Collecting and appraising the evidence
   a. Empirical evidence
      (1) Clinical trials
      (2) Nonexperimental level research
      (3) Systematic reviews/meta-analyses
   b. Nonempirical evidence
      (1) Published reviews
      (2) Published protocols/guidelines
   c. Reading and critically analyzing empirical research for evidence
      (1) Critiquing using the down and dirty approach
         (a) Problem statement
         (b) Literature review
         (c) Theoretical or conceptual framework
         (d) Design
         (e) Ethical considerations
         (f) Instruments
         (g) Sampling
         (h) Data collection
         (i) Data analysis
         (j) Findings/Application
3. Summarizing across the evidence
4. Integrating the evidence with clinical expertise, client preferences and values
   a. Collecting data from clinical experts
   b. Collecting data from the patient
5. Developing the proposed practice change in detail
6. Feasibility issues
   a. Costs
   b. Timeline
   c. Resources
7. Evaluating the practice change
   a. Outcome measures
8. Marketing the practice change
9. Strategies for successful implementation
10. Sustainability of practice change

IDENTIFICATION OF THE CLINICAL PRACTICE PROBLEM

The first step is identification of the clinical practice problem or issue. Frequently, this is the hardest step because it takes much thought and effort to refine the problem statement to develop evidence-based nursing practice projects. If you remember from Chapter 1, identification of the problem is also the first action in designing a research study and can be one of the most difficult steps. For example, maybe the clinical practice problem is patient falls. Falls still constitute a very broad category that requires refinement to develop a good EBNP project. Questions to consider include:

- Do I want to focus on prevention or treatment?
- What population am I focusing on (e.g., elderly, cognitively impaired, physically handicapped)?
- What setting am I interested in (e.g., hospital, long-term care facility, home)?
- What is the current fall rate and when do most of them happen?
- Current fall prevention measures and are they being followed?
- How will I individualize the intervention or practice change (e.g., individual patient fall risk assessment on admission)?

After answering questions such as these, the problem statement in the fall scenario may be "High fall rate of elderly patients on the medical surgical floor related to lack of compliance with fall prevention measures." As you can see, the problem statement can be written very similarly to those you have done for nursing diagnoses statements. You can even use the "as evidenced by" found within the nursing diagnoses framework. Then, your problem statement would read "High fall rate of elderly patients on the medical surgical floor related to lack of compliance with fall prevention measures as evidenced by high current fall rate, lack of documentation of fall prevention measures in the patient's chart, and nurses stating they do not have time to implement the fall prevention protocol."

COLLECTING AND APPRAISING THE EVIDENCE

Step 2 is collecting and appraising the evidence. Both empirical (research) and nonempirical evidence is important to support a practice change. Empirical evidence may include clinical trials, nonexperimental level research, and systematic reviews/meta-analyses. Nonempirical evidence includes published reviews and protocols/guidelines. It is important to discern actual research studies from nonresearch studies. Most nursing journals are very good about directing authors to provide headings so that consumers can find the essential components of a research article. To decide if a particular article is an actual study or not, the first approach would be to examine the abstract. The abstract should contain the problem or purpose statement that should give you a hint about whether this is an actual study or not. Creedon (2006) did an excellent job in the first sentence of the abstract by letting the reader know not only that it was an empirical study, but what type of design was used. Creedon (2006) states: "The primary purpose of this quasi-experimental research is to observe healthcare workers' compliance with hand-hygiene guidelines during patient care in an intensive care unit in Ireland before (pretest) and after (posttest) implementation of a multifaceted hand-hygiene program." The abstract should also include a little about the methods used to conduct the study and study findings and conclusions. It is common in nursing research to find headings throughout the article that incorporate key elements of the research study. Typically, you will be able to find the following sections: background including theoretical framework if there is one, purpose statement (usually the last sentence preceding the methods or procedure sections), methods/procedure section (study design, recruitment and protection of participants, data collecting measures), results, and discussion. If you can find these parts, then you can comfortably assume that you have an article that is reporting original research.

Nonempirical evidence includes published literature reviews, opinion articles, and protocols/guidelines/quality improvement projects. Literature reviews are a review of published research over a particular topic area. Limitations of literature reviews include secondary source of published research, interpretation of the research by someone other than the original researcher, and they may not include all aspects of the topic/issue. Published protocols/evidence-based guidelines/quality improvement projects can provide another form of evidence to synthesize with the empirical research. Just remember, these guidelines were developed for a specific patient population and need to be viewed in that light. Thus, it is advantageous to use them as just one more piece of the evidence but realize that they may or may not translate to the patient or patient population that is your focus.

There are several ways to approach finding the evidence. Electronic databases are an excellent source for finding relevant research. Libraries at universities and many hospitals purchase subscriptions through various vendors such as Ovid, EBSCOhost, Proquest, Gale powersearch, and PubMed. Several of these include MEDLINE, a huge index of medical journal articles, and CINAHL, an index of articles in nursing and allied health journals. Librarians at local universities or at your institution can be invaluable in pointing you in the right direction. A qualified librarian can assist you in deciding what search terms and electronic databases to search to yield the best results. They can also assist you with finding other types of resources both electronically and in other formats that may contribute evidence to your EBNP project.

Sources for evidence-based nursing practice appeared in Table 1-2. There are two main types of literature sources. Primary sources are original, peer-reviewed journal articles, whereas secondary sources are the author's interpretation and comments on primary sources. Since interpretation of study findings can be somewhat subjective, it is good to use primary sources when possible. A discussion on literature searches is found in Chapter 2. As you are finding relevant literature, you will start to see categories of themes emerging. For example, let us consider the problem statement "noncompliance of health-care workers with hand hygiene." Search terms such as "noncompliance and hand hygiene" or "healthcare workers and hand hygiene" or "noncompliance and healthcare workers and hand hygiene" will result in a list of relevant and possibly nonrelevant articles. Sort by topic/focus, such as all of the noncompliance and hand hygiene together and all hand hygiene and healthcare workers together and so on. You may also categorize by research setting or population characteristics (e.g., nurses, doctors, children, older adults).

READING AND CRITICALLY ANALYZING EMPIRICAL RESEARCH

Initially, start with the abstracts to weed out nonrelevant articles. Then, start consuming the research by first skimming the article, particularly paying attention to findings and nursing implications. The next level of reading and analyzing the research involves a more thorough examination and reading of the articles. It may take two or more times through the article before you get a good understanding of the research. Once you have a good idea of what the researchers did, then the next thing to perform is a critical analysis of the study.

To make the critiquing process easier for those who do not have a strong foundation in nursing research but are still expected to consume research and apply the evidence to their practice, I propose a 10-step method to critiquing research. These guidelines are presented in Tables 6-1 and 6-2. This critiquing process will take less than 20 minutes once you have become skilled at using these guidelines. Further detail on each step and complete critique examples are presented in Chapter 6. Those articles deemed credible to use in your evidence-based nursing practice issue will need to be analyzed as a group of studies.

SUMMARIZING ACROSS THE EVIDENCE

This step is very critical to the success of your proposed practice change. Synthesize the findings from the group of empirical research studies you deemed credible. This is done in a very similar way to what is called "content analysis."

Used in this context, content analysis involves examining the findings for recurrent themes across the studies or the majority of studies. Because all research is flawed and has its strengths and limitations, it is dangerous to base a practice change on a single study. However, if you find that multiple studies are proposing the same practice change, then you can start to feel more confident in proposing this change. Now, you need to integrate other forms of evidence collected.

INTEGRATING THE EVIDENCE WITH CLINICAL EXPERTISE AND CLIENT PREFERENCES AND VALUES

The next level of evidence that needs to be synthesized is clinical expertise and patient preferences and values. Expert interviews and current best practice guidelines are resources to assess the clinical expertise available. Experts are persons that have clinical expertise in the topic/problem area of focus. A multidisciplinary approach will ensure a thorough analysis of clinical expertise available. Consider the issue of hand washing noncompliance. Experts not only include nurses, but also infection control personnel, physicians, public health personnel and epidemiologists. To facilitate synthesis and identification of themes across expert interviews, you need to develop a slate of questions for all interviews. Sample interview questions for clients and experts are presented in **Table 5-2**. Interviews and surveys will help to assess individual and/or group client preferences. Without assessing patient needs and preferences, EBNP would just be research utilization. For groups of clients with similar attributes/problems, a survey might be an efficient tool to find out the group's preferences. Clinical expertise comes into play again by the clinician who delivers the actual patient care. It is their responsibility to tailor the EBNP protocol/practice change to the individual client they are providing care to.

DEVELOPING THE PROPOSED PRACTICE CHANGE IN DETAIL

Once all of the evidence is critically analyzed and synthesized, you should have some good ideas for what to propose as an intervention or practice change. For example, if the problem was noncompliance with hand washing by unlicensed staff, and the evidence suggested the primary cause was lack of knowledge, an educational campaign might be your primary focus. Representation by the target population in the development of the practice change is critical for buy-in and success of the change. These individuals can serve as champions for implementation and ultimate success of your project. This step is the point where decisions are made about who will receive the practice change, what will it entail, when will it happen, where will it take place, and how will it take place?

Table 5-2   Sample Interview Questions to Assess Patient Preferences and Clinical Expertise

---

Sample Questions for Patients/Clients

How long have you been dealing with this problem? (You can go ahead and state specifically what the problem is)

What things have you tried to help deal with _____ (problem)? How well have they worked?

What suggestions/treatments have been used by your healthcare provider to help with this problem?

Can you give any examples of what has worked and what has not worked for you personally?

Sample Questions for Experts

Find out credentials, years of experience, and where these years have been spent.

Do not use actual names of experts; use initials or fake names.

What has been your experience with _____ (condition/problem)?

Do you have any successful case studies/scenarios that you can share related to this experience?

What do you think the current best practice is for dealing with this _____ (condition/problem)?

What do you base this answer on? (e.g., research, policies, protocols, providers, etc.)

Is this current best practice you speak of being used in your facility/organization?

If not, why do you think it is not being used? If so, how is it going? How is it being evaluated/outcomes measured?

Would you say that your organization currently uses evidence-based practice? If not, why? If so, can you give an example especially with _____ (condition/problem)?

In the noncompliance with hand washing example, the "who" would be unlicensed staff. The "what" would be the educational campaign to increase knowledge and awareness. Based on the research findings, an outline of the educational content would be developed. Timing of delivery of the education would be the next step to plan. For example, will it be a mandatory educational session for all unlicensed personnel? Will they be paid to attend? How many times will it need to be offered so that all of the target audience can attend? How will compliance with attendance be monitored? Next would be decisions about "where" it will take place. Is there a large enough room close by to the target audience? Are there costs involved in using the location? The "how" of the practice change implementation would include the process leading up to and throughout the actual implementation of the education. Finding representatives from the target audience to champion the cause and to stimulate interest is critical to the success of implementing any practice change. Identification of these individuals occurs early in the process. They are involved in the planning and implementation of the practice change from its inception. Decisions about who will conduct the sessions, length of sessions, availability of refreshments or door prizes, and advertisement and marketing will need to be made.

FEASIBILITY ISSUES

Feasibility issues in implementing evidence-based nursing practice changes include costs, time, and available resources. Each one of these issues is presented below with examples.

Costs/Resources Needed

Budgetary constraints are always an issue for healthcare-related organizations. One of the first things to find out from your organization is how much money they are willing to give to support the proposed practice change. Once you have a plan for the practice change, an itemized budget needs to be developed. Costs may include human resource costs (speaker's salary, target audience paid time to attend) to material resources (printing and paper costs, refreshments, door prizes, advertisement and marketing costs). See **Figure 5-3** for a sample budget. This budget was prepared for an evidence-based nursing practice project on horizontal violence.

Implementation of the proposed practice change of developing the horizontal violence program was financially feasible after taking into consideration issues relating to budget allocations. Expenses were identified for all phases of program implementation and included those for outside resources as well as in-house resources. The estimated total cost of implementing a horizontal violence program for all current nursing staff, new nurses in orientation, competency training materials, computer software, consultant fees, related administrative fees, and personnel expenses was $92,392. This total reflects all costs associated with the first year of program implementation and includes; consultant fees over 4 days, including meals and lodging expenses, initial 4.5 hours of horizontal violence educational training for currently employed nurses, additional orientation training for new nurses in hospital orientation each month, computer software programming fees for the yearly competency training, and the administrative fees such as poster and flyer development and printing and training materials consisting of approximately one 30-minute computerized training session to assess competency in horizontal violence management. Explanation of budget is shown in **Box 5-1**.

Figure 5-3   Sample budget for evidence-based practice projects.

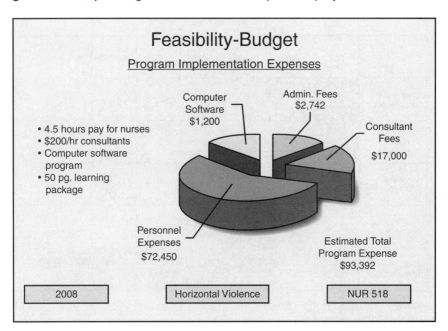

Timeline

A timeline is very useful in ensuring progress towards implementation of the practice change. It also helps organize the details of the planning, implementation, and evaluation of the practice change. A timeline is helpful in keeping all of the players on the same page and communicating completion steps. There are many types of timelines including the Gantt chart (NetMBA Business

Box 5-1   EBNP Budget Allocation Example

1. 460 nurses @ $35/hour × 4.5 hrs initial training = $72,450
2. Consultants @ $200/hour × 40 hrs training over 4 days plus meals and lodging = $17,000
3. 50 pg learning package @0.05/page × 460 = $1150
4. Cover of learning package @0.20/cover × 460 = $92
5. Miscellaneous supplies for educational session and hospital orientation (e.g., posters, flyers, PowerPoint presentation) = $1,500
6. Computer software program = $1,200

TOTAL = $93,392

Figure 5-4   A sample Gantt chart/timeline.

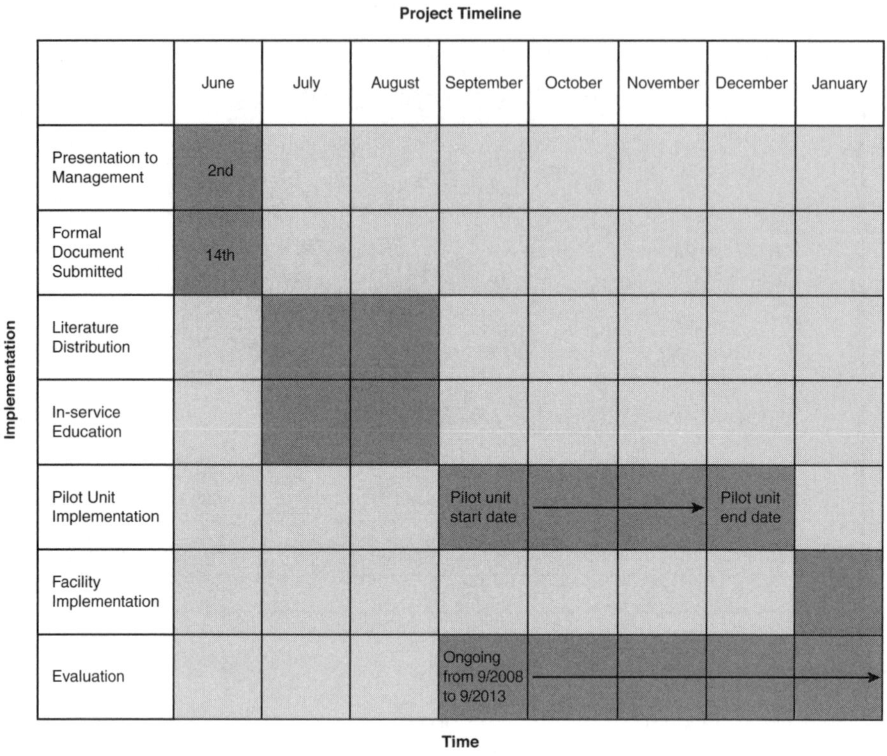

Project Timeline

Implementation	June	July	August	September	October	November	December	January
Presentation to Management	2nd							
Formal Document Submitted	14th							
Literature Distribution								
In-service Education								
Pilot Unit Implementation				Pilot unit start date		→	Pilot unit end date	
Facility Implementation								
Evaluation				Ongoing from 9/2008 to 9/2013				→

Time

Knowledge Center, 2007). A Gantt chart is a type of chart that illustrates a project schedule. Gantt charts illustrate the start and finish dates of the primary activities leading up to completion of the project. Depending on the length of time to project completion, the chart may be broken down by days, weeks, or months. **Figure 5-4** depicts a sample Gantt chart for the hand washing example discussed earlier.

EVALUATING THE PRACTICE CHANGE

To determine the degree of success of the implemented practice change, outcome measures need to be identified. Outcomes must be specific enough so that they are measurable. For example, with the hand washing scenario, immediate outcomes could include attendance at the educational sessions and scoring 90% or better on the knowledge test after the session. Long-term outcomes could include increased rates of hand washing compliance (as compared with baseline) and a decrease in hospital-acquired infections.

MARKETING THE PRACTICE CHANGE

Getting buy-in from the target audience is crucial to the success of any new practice change. As discussed earlier, identifying champions both within the target audience and from other key players that can effect change is imperative for success. In the hand washing example, the target audience is unlicensed personnel. In this case, the evidence-based nursing practice group could include a representation from unlicensed staff, nursing, infection control, and administration.

STRATEGIES FOR SUCCESSFUL IMPLEMENTATION

Several strategies have already been discussed to facilitate a successful EBNP change. Along with having substantial evidence to support your proposed practice change, other strategies include planning, organization, buy-in from stakeholders, recruiting champions for your cause, being realistic regarding available time, money, and resources, and applying principles of change theory to effect change. One popular change theory is Rogers' Diffusion of Innovations. It is a useful framework for understanding social change. The theory deals with dissemination of an innovation (idea, practice, and product) perceived as new by an individual or group of people. It involves a five-step process (Rogers, 2003):

1. Gaining knowledge about the innovation
2. Becoming persuaded about the innovation
3. Decision step of adopting or rejecting the innovation
4. Implementation of putting the innovation to use
5. Confirmation step of reversing the decision or adopting the new innovation

Three characteristics that Rogers identified as central to the adoption decision were the potential user's perception of the benefit to practice, its compatibility with the practice setting and population, and its complexity (Rogers, 2003). Rogers argued for the importance of the user's knowledge on both the how-to and the principles behind the change or innovation. Not only do clinicians need detail about how to implement the practice change, but they also need to understand the underlying theory or framework that explains how the innovation works (Leeman, Jackson, & Sandelowski, 2006).

SUSTAINABILITY OF PRACTICE CHANGE

To sustain or modify the practice change, an evaluation plan should be developed. Identification of measures to be collected, who will be responsible for collecting and how the measures will be analyzed to document level of success will help sustain the practice change. Booster doses (mini-doses of the intervention) over time will also facilitate sustainability of change. For example, back to the hand washing example. Measures of success included participants passing a knowledge posttest with a 90% or better and improved hand washing compliance rates. To sustain this practice, you could have participants do an online education on hand washing and retake the exam each year. Covert observations of the target group (unlicensed personnel) throughout the year on hand washing compliance would also give data to evaluate the success of the practice change. Staff would be made aware that this would be happening but would not know when it occurred in order to reduce the Hawthorn effect (responding differently because they know they are being watched).

THE BIG "SO WHAT?"

- EBNP is a problem-solving approach using current best evidence, clinical expertise, and patient values and preferences to answer a nursing practice problem.
- There are common threads across the major evidence-based practice models that include assessment and identification of the clinical problem, synthesizing the evidence, translating the evidence into a practice change, and implementation and evaluation of the practice change.
- There are 10 steps in evidence-based nursing practice.
- Evidence may include both empirical and nonempirical forms of evidence.
- A clear timeline and itemized costs are necessary for an effective evidence-based nursing practice project.
- Applying principles of planned change is critical to the successful implementation.

REFERENCES

Academic Center for Evidence-Based Practice. (2005). *ACE: Learn about EBP*. Retrieved from http://www.acestar.uthscsa.edu/Learn_model.htm

Creedon, D. (2006). Health care workers' hand decontamination practices: An Irish study. *Clinical Research, 15,* 6–26.

DiCenso, A., Cullum, N., & Ciliska, D. (1998). Implementing evidence-based nursing: Some misconceptions. *Evidence-Based Nursing, 1,* 38–39.

Hermes, B., Deakin, K., Lee, K., & Robinson, S. (2009). Suicide risk assessment: 6 steps to a better instrument. *Journal of Psychosocial Nursing, 47,* 44–49.

Leeman, J., Jackson, B., & Sandelowski, M. (2006). An evaluation of how well research reports facilitate the use of findings in practice. *Journal of Nursing Scholarship, 38,* 171–177.

Melnyk, B., & Fineout-Overholt, E. (2005). *Evidence-based practice in nursing and health care: A guide to best practice.* Philadelphia, PA: Lippincott, Williams, & Wilkins.

NetMBA Business Knowledge Center. (n.d.). *Gantt chart*. Retrieved from http://www.netmba. com/operations/project/gantt/

Newhouse, R., Dearholt, S., Poe, S., Pugh, L., & White, K. (2007). *Johns Hopkins nursing: Evidence-based practice model and guidelines*. Indianapolis, IN: Sigma Theta Tau.

Reavy, K., & Tavernier, S. (2008). Nurses reclaiming ownership of their practice: Implementation of an evidence-based practice model and process. *The Journal of Continuing Education in Nursing, 39*, 166–172.

Rogers, E. M. (2003). *Diffusion of innovations* (5th ed.). New York, NY: Free Press.

Rosswurm, A., & Larrabee, J. H. (1999). A model for change to evidence-based practice. *Image: Journal of Nursing Scholarship, 31*, 317–322.

Rycroft-Malone, J., Seers, K., Titchen, A., Harvey, G., Kitson, A., & McCormack, B. (2004). What counts as evidence in evidence-based practice? *Nursing and Health Care Management and Policy, 47*, 81–90.

Stetler, C. (2001). Updating the Stetler model of research utilization to facilitate evidence-based practice. *Nursing Outlook, 49*, 272–279.

Stevens, K. R. (2004). *ACE Star Model of EBP: Knowledge transformation*. Academic Center for Evidence-Based Practice. San Antonio, TX: The University of Texas Health Science Center. Retrieved from www.acestar.uthscsa.edu

Titler, M. G., Kleiber, C., Steelman, V. J., Rakel, B., Budreau, G., & Everett, L. et al., (2001). The Iowa Model of Evidence-Based Practice to promote quality care. *Critical Care Nursing Clinics of North America, 13*, 497–509.

Tolson, D., Booth, J., & Lowndes, A. (2008). Achieving evidence-based nursing practice: Impact of the Caledonian Development Model. *Journal of Nursing Measurement, 16*, 682–691.

CHAPTER 6

Reading and Critically Analyzing Empirical Research Studies

TEN EASY (OR WILL BECOME EASY) STEPS TO ANALYZING QUANTITATIVE EMPIRICAL RESEARCH

A research critique is a careful, thoughtful examination of a research study, to judge both its strengths and limitations. Following a systematic process is important to obtaining a thorough critique. This chapter will discuss a 10-step process for analyzing quantitative and qualitative research studies. See **Table 6-1** for the 10 steps. As you can see, these steps mirror closely the steps of the research process discussed in Chapter 1.

You might ask, "Why do I need to know how to critically analyze research studies?" If you remember in Chapter 1, the statement was made that, "all research is flawed." If this were not true, there would be no need to analyze research studies. You could just go to the study's findings and recommendations and integrate them into your practice. Even the best of studies has flaws. In nursing, study participants are typically persons living outside of institutions in their communities. It is impossible to control for every possible variable that might influence the results of the study. Therefore, each study has its own inherent weaknesses or limitations.

Analyzing empirical research studies requires considerable critical thinking skills and much practice. The more you practice doing them, the easier it will become. Not only will it become easier, it will take considerably less time to accomplish than when you first started learning how to do them. Table 6-1 lists each step and the specific questions to ask yourself as you analyze each quantitative research study. The table also provides you with a scoring system to categorize the rigor of each study, ranging from excellent to poor. To be considered for use in practice, the study should produce a total score of 35 (fair) or greater. Now, let us take each step and analyze an article published in *Clinical Nursing Research* by this author.

Table 6-1   Ten Steps to Analyzing Quantitative Nursing Research Studies

Step	Specific questions to ask
1. Problem study was designed to solve **(5 points)**	What is the problem statement?
	Is the problem clearly identified by the authors?
	If not, can you create one that fits the study without difficulty?
	Is the problem significant to nursing practice?
2. Research question(s)/ Hypothesis(es) **(5 points)**	What are the research questions and/or hypothesis statements?
	If they were not stated, what would you say the research questions and/or hypothesis statements are?
	What are the study variables (both independent and dependent)?
3. Literature review/ study framework **(5 points)**	Is the literature review sufficient to understand the problem of the study?
	Are the majority of references cited within the last 5 years?
	Can you find a theoretical framework? If so, what is it?
	If a theoretical framework is not present, can you tell from the conceptual framework what connections and relationships are being proposed by the study? If so, what are these relationships? If not, can you infer what the authors are proposing?
	How is the theoretical/conceptual framework used to guide the study?
4. Study design **(5 points)**	What was the quantitative study design used?
	If design is not made explicit by the authors, can you easily determine what design is being used? Based on what rationale?
	In what ways is the design an appropriate one to answer the research question/hypothesis/problem statement?
	Threats to internal and external validity? How are the authors addressing these threats?

Table 6-1   Ten Steps to Analyzing Quantitative Nursing Research Studies
(continued)

Step	Specific questions to ask
5. Sample and setting **(5 points)**	Is the sample appropriate based on design and setting and representativeness of the population?
	What rationale was used to support sample size (i.e., power analysis)?
6. Identification and control of extraneous variables **(5 points)**	What are the main extraneous variables?
	What ways are the authors controlling for them?
7. Study instruments **(5 points)**	What were the instruments (both physiologic and psychological) used to collect data for the study?
	What validity and reliability measures were reported for each?
	Were the selected instruments adequate to measure the study's variables? Why or why not?
8. Data collection methods **(5 points)**	In what ways were the data collection procedures appropriate for the study?
	In what ways were appropriate steps taken to protect the rights of study participants?
	Who approved the study?
	How did the data collection methods match the study design?
9. Data analysis procedures **(5 points)**	In what ways were the data analysis procedures appropriate for the data collected?
	Did the data analysis match the study design? Why or why not?
10. Overall findings/ strengths/limitations **(5 points)**	What were the main findings?
	What were the major strengths of the study?
	What were the major limitations of the study?

Overall ranking of the study—add points across each step for a final score:

Excellent	Good	Fair	Poor
(39–50)	(26–38)	(13–25)	(0–12)

QUANTITATIVE SAMPLE ARTICLE 1

The first article that will be critiqued is an article entitled, "Effects of crossing legs on blood pressure measurement," published in *Clinical Nursing Research*, May 2001. A copy of the published article is reproduced in Appendix 6A at the end of this chapter on pages 113–122.

Here is an example of how this article could be critiqued.

Problem Statement

The problem statement is clearly identified by the authors as follows: "Research is limited on the effect of crossing the leg at the knee during blood pressure measurement" (Keele-Smith & Price-Daniel, 2001). The significance to nursing is clear by the author's opening statements: "Blood pressure monitoring is one of the most commonly used techniques in the diagnosis and treatment of various health care problems. Blood pressure measurement is a crucial tool in determining the existence of hypertension." The authors then discuss the many health problems that hypertension can lead to. **(Score: 4.5)**

Research Question(s)/Hypothesis(es)/Study Variables

The hypothesis for this study was as follows: "It was hypothesized that participants' blood pressure measurements would be higher with legs crossed than with legs uncrossed" (Keele-Smith & Price-Daniel, 2001).

The study variables include the intervention (crossed versus uncrossed legs) as the independent variable and the outcome measure (blood pressure measurements) as the dependent variable. **(Score: 5)**

Literature Review/Background/Framework

The literature review was sufficient to understand the problem of the study. The authors present data to support the numerous factors that may influence blood pressure measurement and results. From talking to food intake to smoking to medications to proper technique; all were discussed. An argument can be made that little research exists on the effects of crossing legs on blood pressure. Only two studies were found examining this issue, and these studies had conflicting findings. Only about half of the references (15) were within the last 5 years from the publication year. No theoretical framework was found. However, the conceptual framework presented links to the importance of accuracy of blood pressure measurements particularly with older adults. There is also a strong link among many factors, including crossing legs and the impact on blood pressure readings. The conceptual framework does a good job of linking the concepts of crossing legs and its impact on blood pressure measurement. **(Score: 4.5)**

Study Design/Sample/Setting

A repeated measures crossover design was used in the study. The design was appropriate to answer the hypothesis statement. Participants either started out with legs crossed or uncrossed. After the first blood pressure measurement, the participants were asked to either cross or uncross their legs depending on which method had not been already used. This method provided a within-subjects comparison of blood pressure measurement with legs crossed and with legs uncrossed.

Threats to internal and external validity were not explicitly stated. However, several strategies were discussed that could decrease these threats. For example, to prevent ordering effects, half of the participants followed one order and the other half followed the reverse order. To prevent inconsistencies in blood pressure measurement, development of standardized protocols and training of data collectors was done. Further, participants were randomly assigned to the two different protocols. All of these strategies would help decrease threats to internal validity such as instrumentation, testing, and selection threats. External validity is limited because only one site was used and the study only included older individuals. However, the sample size was large enough to yield valid findings for this particular sample.

The sample size was appropriate based on a power analysis that resulted in needing a minimum of 98 participants. This study actually had 103 total participants with complete data. The sample came from the population of interest, that is, older adults. Participants were recruited from just two senior citizen centers in the same area. Findings can be generalized at least back to this population. **(Score: 4)**

Identification and Control of Extraneous Variables

Extraneous variables were not explicitly identified. However, from the article, several potential extraneous variables can be identified. Participants who were already diagnosed with hypertension and had not taken their medication or who had peripheral vascular disease were excluded from participating in the study. The researchers, by encouraging participants to use the restroom before data collection and to refrain from other activities prior to participating handled physiologic influences such as caffeine intake, exercise, smoking, and full bladder. The other potential extraneous variable that proved to be one of the major limitations of the study was the socializing/talking that occurred during data collection between the participant and the data collector. **(Score: 4)**

Study Instruments

Blood pressure was measured using a written protocol adapted from the American Heart Association and the National Heart Foundation. Aneroid blood pressure cuffs were used, and each was calibrated to manufacturers' recommendations. Cuff sizes were selected based on the participant's arm circumference. No reliability or validity measures were given for the demographic survey (Keele-Smith & Price-Daniel, 2001). **(Score: 3)**

Data Collection Methods

The researchers randomly assigned participants into treatment groups by selection of either a white or a turquoise marble. Data collectors followed a specific protocol based on marble selection. To reduce the effects of outside stimuli, a quiet room was used for the intervention. Approval to conduct the study was received from both the IRB at New Mexico State University and the Board of Directors that provides oversight at all of the local senior centers in that southern New Mexico city. Written informed consent was also obtained from the participant. A coding system was used to ensure confidentiality and anonymity of the participants. **(Score: 4)**

Data Analysis Procedures

For the primary hypothesis, independent samples T-tests were performed comparing crossed-leg blood pressure readings to uncrossed leg readings. Since blood pressure can be considered interval level data, looking at mean differences between these two groups is appropriate. This statistical analysis also provided the answer to the study's hypothesis. Results indicated that blood pressure was statistically significantly higher when legs were crossed versus uncrossed. Systolic pressure changed by 5.9 mm Hg, and the diastolic pressure changed by 2.97. Even though this was a small change, it was statistically significant. The authors also made the argument that this change, however small, is clinically relevant, particularly in the sample population (Keele-Smith & Price-Daniel, 2001). **(Score: 4)**

Overall Strengths and Limitations

The major strengths and limitations that can be discerned from the article include:

Strengths

- Improves upon prior research examining the same issue
  - Power analysis
  - Equal representation by gender
  - Recommendations by the American Heart Association were followed closely
  - Consistent amount of time to have participants cross and uncross legs

- Random assignment of participants
- Training of data collectors to written protocols
- Support of proposed hypothesis with immediate clinical application
  - Both in education and the work setting, incorporating this protocol into blood pressure measuring would improve validity of measures

Limitations

- Difficulty in keeping seniors quiet during data collection
- Data collected from only two senior citizen centers **(Score: 3.5)**

Total Score: 41.5 (Good)

QUANTITATIVE SAMPLE ARTICLE 2

The second article that will be critiqued is an article entitled, "Evaluation of individually tailored interventions on exercise adherence," published in *Western Journal of Nursing Research 25*(6), 623–640. A copy of the published article is reproduced in Appendix 6B at the end of this chapter on pages 123–140.

Here is an example of how this article could be critiqued.

Problem Statement

The problem statement is clearly identified by the authors as follows: "Although the benefits of exercise are abundant, as little as 30% of the adult population in the United States remains committed to a regular exercise regimen" (Keele-Smith & Leon, 2003). The authors go on to say that motivation is a key factor in predicting adherence, but those motives vary by individual and have been difficult to measure. The significance to nursing is clear by the author's opening statement that "practitioners need to know these motives when designing exercise interventions." **(Score: 5)**

Research Question(s)/Hypothesis(es)/Study Variables

The hypothesis was easy to find and even had its own heading. The authors state, "Participants in the education plus monitoring group will have a greater number of consistent exercisers and higher exercise motivation scores than will those in the monitoring-only group. Participants in the education plus monitoring group will have greater overall weight loss and decrease in percentage of body fat measurements than will those in the monitoring-only group. Consistent exercisers will score higher than will inconsistent exercisers on exercise motivation scores" (Keele-Smith & Leon, 2003).

The study variables include the intervention (education plus monitoring or monitoring-only) as the independent variable and the outcome measure (frequency and duration of exercise, weight, percentage of body fat, exercise motivation scores) as the dependent variables. **(Score: 5)**

Literature Review/Background/Framework

The literature review was sufficient to understand the problem of the study. The authors present data to support the numerous factors that may affect exercise, including benefits and barriers. They also give the reader a background regarding exercise motivation and individual motives for exercising as it relates to reversal theory. Reversal theory provided the theoretical framework for this study. Reversal theory is described briefly and then discussed in light of identifying individual exercise motives. The authors make the point that no research has been done using reversal theory as a guide in designing individual exercise interventions (Keele-Smith & Leon, 2003). **(Score: 5)**

Study Design/Sample/Setting

Study design is the first thing discussed under the methodology of the study. An experimental pretest–posttest design was used with participants being randomly assigned into the two treatment groups. The design was appropriate to answer the hypothesis statement since the purpose of this study was to test an intervention.

Threats to internal and external validity were not explicitly stated. However, several strategies were discussed that could decrease these threats. For example, to prevent inconsistencies in outcome measurements, development of standardized protocols and training of data collectors was done. Further, participants were randomly assigned to the two different protocols. Data collection instruments had acceptable levels of validity and reliability. All of these strategies would help decrease threats to internal validity such as instrumentation, testing, and selection threats. External validity is limited due to the fact that only one site (university) was used. However, based on a power analysis, the sample size was large enough to yield valid findings for this particular sample. One threat to validity that was not discussed was the possibility of contamination across treatment groups. Since participants all came from the same university, it is highly possible that contact with other participants could have occurred.

The sample size was 149 adults, which was more than the required minimum of 126 participants based on the power analysis. The sample came from the population of interest, that is, faculty, staff, and students at a local university. **(Score: 4.5)**

Identification and Control of Extraneous Variables

Extraneous variables were not explicitly identified. However, from the article, several potential extraneous variables can be identified. Females primarily made up the sample, and overall the sample was highly educated. Overall, the sample was healthy and young. Generalization of study findings beyond the study site should be done with caution. **(Score: 4)**

Study Instruments

Weight and body fat were measured using the TANITA Body Fat Monitor/Scale TBF-612. Description of the scale, how it was administered, and measures of reliability (comparing the scale with underwater weighing) were provided. For the EMQ, the authors give a complete description by sharing format, scoring, and example items for each subscale. Cronbach's alphas, a measure of internal consistency reliability, was given for all subscales prior to and for this study. For this study, they ranged from 0.70 to 0.95. The authors provide support of convergent and discriminant validity by describing predicted relationships between the EMQ and the Exercise Motivation Inventory. They also present a detailed table depicting actual correlations for the reader to discern. No validity or reliability measures were given for the weekly exercise questionnaire completed by the interview with participants. **(Score: 4.5)**

Data Collection Methods

Since this was an experimental pretest–posttest design, outcome measures (body fat, weight, motivation scores, level of exercise) were collected at the beginning and at the end of the study. Researchers did random assignment into treatment groups. Data collectors received the same training sessions to ensure consistency of protocol and measurement of outcome variables. The treatment (a written individualized exercise prescription), developed by the principal investigator, was consistently reinforced weekly by the student data collectors. However, the researchers do not include much detail about what the actual interventions included. Approval to conduct the study was received from the Human Participants Review Committee at the university where the principal investigator is a faculty member. Written informed consent was also obtained from the participants. Participants were also informed about consulting with their healthcare provider regarding safety and any risks in participating. **(Score: 4)**

Data Analysis Procedures

The data analysis procedures were appropriate for the data collected and for the study design. Based on the experimental design, tests were done to determine differences on outcomes from the beginning to the end of the study. For continuous data, independent sample T-tests were conducted on between-group mean differences, and paired samples T-tests were performed on within-group mean differences between weight, body fat, and motivation scores. For categorical data, nonparametric tests were used (e.g., cross-tabs procedure). **(Score: 5)**

Overall Strengths and Limitations

The major strengths and limitations that can be discerned from the article include:

Strengths

- Experimental level design
- Randomization of sample into treatment groups
- Adequate sample size
- Theoretically grounded
- Consistent exercisers had higher motivation scores when compared to inconsistent exercisers
- More participants were exercising regularly in the education plus monitoring group than in the monitoring group only after the study intervention
- Low attrition rate

Limitations

- Limited generalizability since only one setting used
- Short time period (5 weeks) given the outcome measures (weight, body fat)
- Possible contamination between treatment groups if participants talked to other participants both within and across groups **(Score: 4)**

Total Score: 46 (Excellent)

TEN STEPS IN ANALYZING QUALITATIVE RESEARCH STUDIES

The next type of empirical research we need to know how to analyze is the qualitative research study. Qualitative research can be analyzed using most of the same steps you just learned with quantitative research studies. However, many of the specific questions that need to be asked are not the same since qualitative research serves a different purpose. Let us take a couple of published qualitative research studies, just like we did with quantitative research, and analyze them using the steps and questions depicted in **Table 6-2.**

QUALITATIVE SAMPLE ARTICLE 1

The first qualitative article that will be critiqued is an article entitled, "Transforming the death sentence: Elements of hope in women with advanced ovarian

---

Table 6-2   Ten Steps to Analyzing Qualitative Nursing Research Studies

Step	Specific questions to ask
1. Problem study was designed to solve **(5 points)**	What is the problem the study was conducted to resolve?
	Why is the problem an important one for nursing practice?
2. Purpose statement/ Research question(s) **(5 points)**	What is the purpose of the study?
	What rationale do the authors give to support a qualitative approach?
	What is the research question? If it is not stated, what would you say the research question is?
	Would you say that the question is stated broadly enough for a qualitative study?
3. Literature review/ Study framework **(5 points)**	Does the particular qualitative method used call for a literature review and/or conceptual framework prior to initiating fieldwork?
	If so, is the review sufficiently comprehensive?
	Are major concepts identified and defined?
	If a literature review is appropriate only after data collection, does the researcher outline a process for accomplishing this?
	If bracketing assumptions are an important component of the qualitative method selected, is this process explained?
	Are the majority of references cited within the last 5 years?
4. Study design **(5 points)**	What was the qualitative study design used?
	If the design is not made explicit by the authors, can you easily determine what design is being used? Based on what rationale?
	In what ways is the design an appropriate one to answer the research question or purpose statement?
5. Sample and setting **(5 points)**	Are the sample's characteristics (demographics, size) appropriate based on design and setting? Rationale for answer?
6. Identification and control for threats to rigor **(5 points)**	Threats to rigor? How are the authors addressing these threats?

(continued)

Table 6-2   Ten Steps to Analyzing Qualitative Nursing Research Studies (continued)

Step	Specific questions to ask
7. Instruments used to collect data **(5 points)**	What instruments were used to collect data? Appropriateness of these instruments based on study design?
8. Data collection methods **(5 points)**	In what ways were the data collection procedures appropriate for the study? In what ways were appropriate steps taken to protect the rights of study participants? Who approved the study? How did the data collection methods match the study design? Does the researcher outline a plan for keeping data organized and retrievable? Explain answer.
9. Data analysis procedures **(5 points)**	In what ways were the data analysis procedures appropriate for the data collected? Did the data analysis match the study design? Why or why not? What evidence is there that data saturation was achieved?
10. Overall findings/ strengths/limitations **(5 points)**	What were the main findings? What were the major strengths of the study? What were the major limitations of the study?

Overall ranking of the study—add points across each step for a final score:

Excellent	Good	Fair	Poor
(39–50)	(26–38)	(13–25)	(0–12)

cancer," published in *Oncology Nursing Forum*, *34*, 2007, E70-81. A copy of the published article is reproduced in Appendix 6C at the end of this chapter on pages 141–170.

Here is an example of how this article could be critiqued.

Problem Study Was Designed to Solve

The problem was clearly identified by the author. The problem that this study is trying to address is quality of life concerns of women with advanced ovarian cancer. Further, limited research has addressed hope in women with ovarian cancer and hope and quality of life concerns associated with long-term treatment (Reb, 2007). Significance of the problem was not explicit but easy to determine. The problem is significant for nursing practice since nurses have frequent contact with women with advanced ovarian cancer as they seek long-term medical treatment. Nurses are also usually at the forefront with addressing patient concerns such as quality of life and dealing with advanced cancer on a daily basis. **(Score: 4)**

Purpose Statement/Research Question(s)

The purpose of the study as stated by Reb (2007) was to describe the experience of hope in women with advanced ovarian cancer. The author does not provide a specific rationale to support a qualitative approach. However, the purpose is to describe the *experience* of women with advanced ovarian cancer. The purpose matches the purpose of a qualitative approach; that is, to describe life experiences and give them meaning. The fact that limited research exists over this topic is also support for a qualitative exploratory design. The author cited no specific research questions. However, the purpose statement can be considered broad enough for a qualitative study. **(Score: 4)**

Literature Review/Study Framework

The qualitative method used in this study is a modified version of grounded theory. The author does a good job by pointing out that a comprehensive literature review is not done initially so that the substantive theory emerges from the participant data. Once the theory is sufficiently developed, the relevant literature is integrated (Reb, 2007). However, a brief literature review and conceptual orientation is given to give the reader perspective into the issue. For example, prior research to support the problem of ovarian cancer and issues related to quality of life are presented at the beginning of the study. An argument is made about the lack of research available that describes the experience of hope in women with this advanced cancer. The conceptual orientation for this study is based on symbolic interactionism and constructivist paradigms. The author gives definitions of each as it relates to this study. Bracketing is not discussed. **(Score: 3)**

Study Design

As mentioned earlier, a modified version of grounded theory was used. The author states that this method was appropriate for the topic since grounded theory is process oriented and seeks to discover theoretical explanations when little information is available (Reb, 2007). However, the author does not state how the methodology was modified. **(Score: 4)**

Sample and Setting

The sample was purposive and included 20 women with the majority diagnosed with stage III or greater ovarian cancer. Based on the Sandelowski (1995) rule of thumb of 30 observations/participants for grounded theory, the sample size was a little small. However, it is important to note that data saturation occurred after just 17 focused interviews. Interviews were done in natural settings such as the participant's home, workplace, and even a local restaurant. **(Score: 5)**

Identification and Control for Threats to Rigor

Trustworthiness or rigor of the data was addressed by close adherence to the methodology and addressing criteria for trustworthiness (credibility, transferability, dependability, and confirmability). Examples were given to support this statement. For example, experts in grounded theory methodology audited several transcripts and followed the researcher's decision trail. In addition, member-checking was done by one participant who commented on the findings during the final stages of analysis. **(Score: 5)**

Instruments Used to Collect Data

A personal data form and a focused interview guide were used to collect data. Demographic information was collected on the personal data form, and the interview guide included open-ended questions about women's experiences of hope. These instruments were appropriate for grounded theory since they were based on the concept of hope and input from clinical nurse experts and doctorally prepared nurses with expertise in grounded theory methodology. **(Score: 5)**

Data Collection Methods

After informed consent was obtained, each participant completed a personal data form prior to interview. Each participant came up with her own pseudonym as an identifier. Interviews that lasted 1.5 to 2 hours were transcribed verbatim from the tapes. Data were collected until saturation occurred, which was after just 17 interviews. Three additional interviews were done just to ensure no new information emerged. Data collection methods used by this researcher are rigorous and follow the grounded theory methodology. Permission to do the study was obtained by all relevant review boards. Patient consent was obtained, and the patient's provider did screening. The only discussion on how the data was organized and retrieved was that the interviews were transcribed verbatim and that line-by-line coding was done using ethnograph software program. **(Score: 4)**

Data Analysis Methods

Constant comparative method is the appropriate data analysis to use with grounded theory. Line-by-line coding of transcribed interviews was done to identify key concepts. An inductive approach was used going from codes to categories with the goal of identifying the core variable. Theoretical coding was used to conceptualize how the substantive codes related to each other. Memos were used to focus the categories. The author states that data saturation occurred after the 17th interview. **(Score: 5)**

Overall Strengths and Limitations

Transforming the death threat emerged as the core variable. Three phases of trajectory were shock, aftershock, and rebuilding. Communication by the healthcare provider and the individual's own spirituality influenced hope and the participant's ability to transform the death sentence. Support and perceived control also emerged as key dimensions of the core variable. Knowledge related to community support services may also increase feelings of control in these women.

Strengths of the study include rigor in design and methodology and identifying practical nursing implications that can be used with women with advanced ovarian cancer. Identification of vulnerable points of distress for this sample of women is also helpful for healthcare providers to target specific interventions during this time to reduce associated distress and anxiety.

The major limitation as identified by the researcher is the lack of a longitudinal approach and using more than one interview over time. Rapport and trust takes time and having extended contact over time may increase the depth of women's experiences and hope. **(Score: 5)**

Total Score: 44 (Good)

QUALITATIVE SAMPLE ARTICLE 2

The second qualitative article that will be critiqued is an article entitled, "A place to be yourself: Empowerment from the client's perspective," published in *Image, Journal of Nursing Scholarship*, *25*, 1993, 297–303. A copy of the published article is reproduced in Appendix 6D at the end of this chapter on pages 171–185.

Here is an example of how this article could be critiqued.

Problem Study Was Designed to Solve

The problem was not clearly identified in the study. From the opening paragraphs of the study, it appears that mental health staff at the research setting wanted to know the impact of the drop-in center that was being overseen by a client board of seven directors. However, they did not have the time to study the effects in detail, so they welcomed outside help from this doctoral student group. Community-based mental health centers are essential for providing a comprehensive, community-based program of care for behavioral health clients. **(Score: 3)**

Purpose Statement/Research Question(s)

The authors provide two research questions as follows:

1. What is the clients' perspective of the factors that make the drop-in center successful?
2. Do clients perceive themselves as having more power to make decisions than they had before the drop-in center was started? **(Score: 5)**

Literature Review/Study Framework

The authors present the conceptual framework thoroughly and clearly for this study. They present critical background information to support the need for this study, including key legislation that has influenced mental health with the goal of increased consumer input. The setting for this study is a client-run drop-in center for community-based behavioral health clients. This study was based on a prior full-scale ethnography of a group of chronically mentally ill clients that studied the difficulties experienced as they dealt with everyday issues. The qualitative method used was a focused ethnography following the principles of an emergent design. As with most qualitative methods, most of the literature review was done after data analysis to reduce preconceived biases. The last sentence in the data analysis section states that the literature on empowerment was reviewed for relevance after the data analysis had been completed. Bracketing is not discussed nor is the rationale for doing the majority of literature review after data collection. The majority of references (19 out of 47) are within 5 years of the date of study publication. Several of the older references are critical to providing a foundation for the ethnography methods used and for background on the community mental health movement. **(Score: 5)**

Study Design

A focused ethnography was used to describe the client's experiences at the mental health drop-in center. The authors do a good job of providing the rationale for this choice. They share that "the goal of ethnography is to grasp the subject's point of view." This design is appropriate to answer the research questions since both initial questions are seeking the "client's perspective." **(Score: 5)**

Sample and Setting

The sample only included 16 informants (12 clients and 4 professional staff). This is small even for a qualitative study since the rule of thumb as provided by Sandelowski (1995) is 30 to 50 interviews for an ethnography. The setting (Prairie Place) was appropriate for the population of interest since the researchers were interested in how the participants perceived the client-run drop-in center. **(Score: 3)**

Identification and Control for Threats to Rigor

To avoid threats to rigor such as observer bias, data and investigator triangulation was used. Peer debriefing and member-checking with selected informants was also used. **(Score: 5)**

Instruments Used to Collect Data

Instruments used to collect data were not described clearly. From reading the article, it can be determined that paper and pencil were used to write detailed field notes of the interviews and observations. Documents such as relevant newspaper articles, agency brochures, letters from the clients to the board and client-made posters/buttons were data sources. **(Score: 4)**

Data Collection Methods

Data collection included interviews, participant observation, and document review. These are all common data collection strategies with qualitative methodology. The human subjects committee approved the study, and the purpose was explained at a client board meeting. To reduce intrusiveness, audio, and videotaping were not used. The authors did not include a discussion on how each participant gave informed consent.

Detailed field notes were transcribed as soon as possible after the interviews. Participant-observations were written up as soon as possible after the observations. No other description of how data was organized is given. **(Score: 3)**

Data Analysis Methods

Data were analyzed using Spradley's recommended method. Each researcher coded separately their own field notes, and then the data were pooled into informant domains. Group consensus led to the merging of these 36 domains into 5 major domains with empowerment identified as the dominant theme. Data saturation is not discussed. **(Score: 3)**

Overall Strengths and Limitations

Four domains of the process of empowerment emerged from the data. The fifth domain represented the effects of empowerment and its meaning for individual clients. In the process of data analysis, a definition of empowerment was developed. Each domain's characteristics were described along with participant examples. Another unique finding was the development of a model of empowerment. From the client's perspective, empowerment meant more participation and more choices for them. It also meant support given to one another and an ability to negotiate outcomes with staff.

Limitations were not clearly stated. However, ethnography usually takes a much longer period of time than 5 weeks. Further, the sample size was small even for qualitative methodology. No evidence of data saturation was found, leaving the reader to wonder about the threat of premature closure and holistic fallacy. **(Score: 3)**

Total Score: 39 (Fair)

THE BIG "SO WHAT?"

- All research is flawed. Therefore, it is important to be able to analyze critically the strengths and weaknesses of a research study.
- There are 10 easy steps to analyzing either quantitative or qualitative research studies.
- The more you practice, the easier the critiquing process will become.
- A score of 35 (Fair) or better is needed for consideration for use in practice.

REFERENCES

Connelly, L., Keele, B., Kleinbeck, S., Schneider, J., & Cobb, A. (1993). A place to be yourself: Empowerment from the client's perspective. *Image, Journal of Nursing Scholarship, 25,* 297–303.

Keele-Smith, R., & Price-Daniel, C. (2001). Effects of crossing legs on blood pressure measurement. *Clinical Nursing Research, 10,* 202–213.

Keele-Smith, R., & Leon, T. (2003). Evaluation of individually tailored interventions on exercise adherence. *Western Journal of Nursing Research, 25,* 623–651.

Reb, A. (2007). Transforming the death sentence: Elements of hope in women with advanced ovarian cancer. *Oncology Nursing Forum, 34,* E70–E81.

Sandelowski, M. (1995). Focus on qualitative methods: Sample size in qualitative research. *Research in Nursing & Health, 18,* 179–183.

Effects of Crossing Legs on Blood Pressure Measurement

REBECCA KEELE-SMITH
New Mexico State University

CECILIA PRICE-DANIEL
MAJ, Army Nurse Corps

The purpose of this study was to determine if blood pressure measurement is affected by the leg crossed at the knee as compared with feet flat on the floor in a well-senior population. Participants (N = 110) either had their blood pressure measured with feet flat first and then crossed or the reverse of this. Results indicate that blood pressure was significantly higher when legs were crossed versus uncrossed. Systolic pressure changed by 5.9 mmHg, from 127.32 to 133.24, whereas diastolic pressure changed by 2.97, from 72.54 to 75.52. There were no significant differences between those who had their blood pressure measured first with their legs crossed versus uncrossed or between those with and without hypertension. Instructing patients to keep feet flat on the floor during blood pressure measurement is an important nursing intervention that can contribute to the accurate measurement, interpretation, and treatment of a patient's health condition.

Authors' Note: The views expressed in this article are those of the author and do not reflect the official policy or position of the Department of Army, the Department of Defense, or the U.S. government. We would like to thank the following M.S.N. students from New Mexico State University for their help in designing this study, recruiting participants, and collecting data: Elisabeth P. Christeson, R.N., B.S.N.; Robert Navarrette, R.N., B.S.N.; Trinette Radasa, R.N., B.S.N.; Mary Beth Fuller-Manning, R.N., B.S.N.; and Ann McCaul Buckley, R.N., B.S.N.

Blood pressure monitoring is one of the most commonly used techniques in the diagnosis and treatment of various health care problems. Blood pressure measurement is a crucial tool in determining the existence of hypertension. Hypertension can lead to congestive heart failure, arteriosclerosis, and thrombi, which may cause heart attack or stroke. The determination of hypertension is especially important in the elderly population. There are numerous

From "Effects of crossing legs on blood pressure management," by R. Keele-Smith, & C. Price–Daniel, 2001, *Clinical Nursing Research, 10*(2), 202–213. Copyright 2001 by Sage Publications. Reprinted with permission.

physiological factors related to the aging process (e.g., rigidity of blood vessels, exaggerated effects from meals, sodium intake, and full bladder) that make hypertension more serious in this population (Campbell & Mckay, 1994; Campbell, Hogan, & Mckay, 1994; Sadowski & Redeker, 1996). Among America's elderly population, 50% have diagnosed hypertension (Sadowski & Redeker, 1996). All efforts should be made to eliminate errors in measuring blood pressure. Although some guidelines for accurately measuring a patient's blood pressure include instructing the patient to keep their feet flat on the floor, research is limited on the effect of crossing the leg at the knee during blood pressure measurement. This study was initiated to determine if blood pressure measurement is affected when a leg is crossed at the knee as compared with feet flat on the floor in a well-senior population.

BACKGROUND

Numerous factors influence an individual's blood pressure measurement. Talking immediately before and during blood pressure measurement and the "white coat effect" have been studied by Le Paullieur et al. (1996, 1998) and Parati et al. (1998). Findings are that these factors can significantly increase blood pressure readings.

Inconsistency in blood pressure technique by health care providers can also affect the validity and reliability of blood pressure measurement. In a study by Gillespie and Curzio (1998), on assessing staff knowledge, it was determined that 74% of hospital nurses were unable to determine blood pressure measurement properly. Frankel (1999) researched the techniques used by 2nd-year medical students. Participants received extensive training in proper blood pressure technique during their first year of medical school. Findings showed that 75% displayed an improper technique. Factors such as proper cuff size, proper cuff placement, taking into account interarm differences, and difficulty in assessing Kortokoff sounds affect blood pressure measurement (Anderson & Maloney, 1994; Campbell, Hogan, & Mckay, 1994; Campbell, McKay, Chockalingam, & Fodor, 1994a, 1994c; Hollander & Singer, 1997; Perloff et al., 1993; Torrance & Serginson, 1996). Bardwell (1995); Baker and Ende (1995); Torrance (1997); and Netea, Smits, Lenders, and Thien (1998, 1999) discussed the importance of arm position, arm support, back support, and body position. Netea et al. (1999) studied arm position and determined that false elevated systolic and diastolic readings can result when arm position is below the right atrial level.

There are many physiological influences on blood pressure measurement. Moriera, Fuchs, Moraes, Bredemeier, and Duncan (1998); Campbell, Hogan, and McKay (1994); and Campbell and McKay (1994) discussed some of these factors. Influences such as proximity of alcohol and food intake before blood pressure measurement, the effect of bowel and bladder distention, caffeine intake, proximity of exercise prior to the measurement, smoking, and medications can result in a skewed blood pressure reading.

One factor only recently researched is the effect of crossing legs on blood pressure measurement. The physiologic mechanism for the rise in blood pressure with leg crossing is a translocation of blood volume from the dependent vascular beds to the thoracic compartment. Case reports have documented the usefulness of leg crossing as a physical maneuver to maintain blood pressure in orthostatic hypotension (van Lieshout, ten Harkel, & Wieling, 1992).

Few articles were found that specifically examined the effects of crossing legs on blood pressure. Cooper (1992), Rudy (1986), and Hill and Grim (1991) recommended that patients keep both feet flat on the floor during blood pressure measurement. Blood pressure research does not typically control for leg position as a measurement variable (Jamieson et al., 1990). Foster-Fitzpatrick, Ortiz, Sibilano, Marcantonio, and Braun (1999) studied the specific effects of crossing legs on blood pressure measurement. A convenience sample of 100 hypertensive male persons was selected from various outpatient clinics in an inner-city acute-care veteran's hospital. The first 50 participants positioned their feet flat on the floor while their blood pressure was measured. After 3 minutes, the blood pressure was measured again with the participant's leg crossed at the knee. The procedure was reversed for the second 50 participants. Results of the repeated measures analysis of variance were significant with the crossed-leg position. Systolic pressure increased on an average of 9.45 mmHg, and diastolic pressure increased by 3.7 mmHg. Peters, Binder, and Campbell (1999) had similar findings in a crossover design using 50 healthy volunteers and 53 hypertensive participants. Systolic blood pressure increased on an average of 8.1 mmHg, and diastolic blood pressure increased 4.5 mmHg in participants with hypertension who crossed their legs during the procedure. Crossing legs increased systolic pressure by 2.5 mmHg in the healthy volunteers but had little effect on diastolic blood pressure.

Due to this limited research and somewhat conflicting findings, this study was developed to add to the body of research examining the effects of crossing legs on blood pressure measurement. It was hypothesized that participants' blood pressure measurements would be higher with legs crossed than with legs uncrossed.

METHOD

A repeated measures crossover design was used with the independent variable being the crossing of one leg. The dependent variable was the blood pressure measurement before and after one leg is crossed.

Table 1   Blood Pressure Protocol

---

1. Sit participant in a chair with arms bared and supported at heart level.
2. Begin measurement after 5 minutes of rest.
3. Select appropriate cuff size. Bladder should be at least 80% of the arm's circumference.
4. Center cuff bladder over the artery about 2 cm above the bend in the elbow.
5. While feeling the radial pulse, note the point of inflation where pulse disappears.
6. Wait 30 seconds. Using stethoscope auscultating over the brachial artery, inflate cuff to 30 mmHg above the palpated systolic pressure.
7. Release the air in the cuff at a rate of 2 mmHg per second.
8. The first appearance of sound (Korotkoff sounds, Phase 1) is used to define the systolic blood pressure. The disappearance of sound (Korotkoff sounds, Phase 5) is used to define diastolic blood pressure.

Blood Pressure Measurement

Blood pressure measurements were performed and recorded by six registered nurses enrolled in a graduate nursing research class at a local university. A written protocol (see **Table 1**) for taking blood pressure was adapted from the American Heart Association and the National Heart Foundation (Anderson & Maloney, 1994; Joint National Committee VI, 1997). Aneroid blood pressure cuffs were used and each was calibrated according to manufacturers' instructions. Cuff sizes were selected on the basis of the participant's arm circumference. Practice sessions were held using the blood pressure protocol to ensure a proper and consistent technique among nurse researchers.

Procedures

Participants, without looking, selected a marble from a basket containing 50 white and 50 turquoise marbles. Participants were randomly assigned to either the turquoise-marble protocol or the white-marble protocol based on their selection of marbles. After a consent form and a demographic form were completed, participants were escorted to a quiet room. Researchers followed the appropriate protocol depending on the color of the marble that participants selected. The turquoise-marble protocol had participants sitting with feet flat on the floor, relaxing for 3 minutes. Blood pressure was measured at the end of the 3-minute period. Participants were then asked to cross one leg (the leg of comfort) over the knee and hold this position for 3 minutes. Blood pressure measurement was repeated at the end of this 3-minute period. The white-marble protocol was just the reverse of the turquoise-marble protocol. The purpose of this reverse ordering for part of the sample was to reduce the possibility of ordering effects that could skew the results.

Participants

Participants for this study were seniors attending activities at two local senior citizen centers. They were recruited by word of mouth and informational flyers at local senior centers. Based on a power analysis using an effect size of .40, a power of .80, and an alpha of .05, a minimum of 98 participants was needed to achieve an adequate level of power (Cohen, 1988). Participants could be normotensive or hypertensive. To reduce the risk of increasing blood pressure to an unsafe level when legs were crossed, participants were excluded if they were taking antihypertensives and had not taken their medication the day of the data collection. Other exclusionary criteria included having the diagnosis of peripheral vascular disease, lower leg amputations, surgery within the past 2 weeks, inability to cross legs, or any other condition that would decrease their ability to cross their legs safely.

Ethical Considerations

Participants were informed that participation was voluntary and that they may withdraw from the study at anytime. Approval to conduct the study was obtained through the Human Subjects Committee at New Mexico State University where the primary investigator is presently a faculty member and from the Board of Directors at Munson Senior Center, all located in the same southern New Mexico city. Written informed consent was obtained from each participant. No risks were expected, but participants were informed that, if necessary, referrals would be made to their primary care physician or local hospital. Benefits would include improvement of patient care through a more accurate assessment of blood pressure. Confidentiality and anonymity were ensured by using a coding system of numbers and not using any participant-identifying information on any data collection instruments.

RESULTS

One hundred and ten seniors participated in the study. Seven participants were excluded; 6 participants were excluded because they had not taken their blood pressure medication on the day of measurement and 1 participant had a seizure during data collection. Therefore, there was a total of 103 participants available for data analysis. Ages ranged from 50 to 92 years, with a mean age of 70.8. Fifty-two participants were female and 51 participants were male. Sixty participants were non-Hispanic White (58.3%), 28 (27.2%) were Hispanic, and 2 (12.6%) were Black. Thirteen participants had missing data for this category. There was almost an equal number of participants in each

Table 2   _t_ Tests for Paired Samples Comparing Blood Pressures With Legs Crossed With Blood Pressures With Legs Uncrossed

	Paired _t_ Test			Mean		Standard Deviation	
	N	t	p	Crossed	Uncrossed	Crossed	Uncrossed
Systolic blood pressures	103	7.22	< .001	133.24	127.32	18.44	18.43
Diastolic blood pressures	103	5.04	< .001	75.52	72.54	10.37	11.71

educational background, ranging from 27 (26.2%) with less than a high school education to 28 (27.2%) with a college degree. A little over half of the sample (51.5%) had at least some college or a college degree. The majority of the participants (54.4%) rated their health status as good. Twenty-eight (27.2%) participants rated their health as fair, and 1 one rated his or her health as poor. There were 49 participants who stated they were being treated for hypertension and 54 who were not.

To test for order effects, the crossed-leg systolic and diastolic blood pressures for the turquoise-marble group were compared with the crossed-leg

Table 3   Results of Independent Sample _t_ Tests Comparing Blood Pressures Between Those Who Have Hypertension Versus Those Who Do Not

	_t_ Test			Mean		Standard Deviation	
	N	t	p	High	Not High	High	Not High
Systolic blood pressure with legs crossed	103	1.34	.182	135.80	130.93	2.97	2.16
Diastolic blood pressure with legs crossed	103	0.76	0.452	76.33	74.78	10.70	10.10
Systolic blood pressure with legs uncrossed	103	1.22	.227	129.63	125.22	21.44	15.09
Diastolic blood pressure with legs uncrossed	103	0.06	.955	72.61	72.48	12.03	11.53

systolic and diastolic blood pressures for the white-marble group. Independent sample *t* tests were nonsignificant, indicating that order effects were not present. Crossed-leg and uncrossed-leg blood pressure measurements for each group were then combined and paired sample *t* tests were performed between them. Results indicate that blood pressure was significantly higher when legs were crossed versus uncrossed. This was true for both the systolic and diastolic blood pressure. Systolic pressure changed by 5.9 mmHg, from 127.32 to 133.24, whereas diastolic pressured changed by 2.97, from 72.54 to 75.52. See **Table 2** for specific results.

To compare blood pressure measurement between those who stated they were being treated for hypertension and those who did not have hypertension, independent sample *t* tests were performed. No significant differences between blood pressures were found whether the participants' legs were crossed or uncrossed. See results of these tests in **Table 3**.

DISCUSSION

Only limited research has examined the effects of crossing legs on blood pressure. Foster-Fitzpatrick et al. (1999) specifically examined the effects of crossed legs on blood pressure and found that it increased significantly with the crossed-leg position. This study not only supports the findings of Foster-Fitzpatrick et al. but measures to improve validity and reliability were added to the current study. A power analysis was conducted to determine the appropriate sample size needed to achieve an adequate level of power that resulted in a larger sample size than the prior study. The study sample equally represented men and women, which is an improvement over prior research. There was an equal representation of both normatensive and hypertensive participants within the sample. Zero-calibrated aneroid sphygmomanometers were used as recommended by the American Heart Association (Joint National Committee VI, 1997). A consistent length of time was used for participants to have their legs crossed before the blood pressure was taken. Having legs crossed for inconsistent periods before obtaining measurements could have confounded the results. To improve the strength of the design, random assignment was used to determine which protocol participants received during data collection. Furthermore, training sessions were held for data collectors to ensure consistency of the blood pressure measurement technique. All data collectors followed written protocols that had been pilot tested at an earlier time. To reduce the number of physiological influences on blood pressure measurement, participants were encouraged to use the restroom if needed and to refrain from caffeine intake, exercise, and smoking prior to data collection.

Contrary to Peters et al.'s study (1999), there were no differences found in blood pressures whether the legs were crossed or uncrossed between those who were being treated for hypertension and those who were not. Blood pressure measurement was significantly higher when legs were crossed versus uncrossed for both groups.

The biggest limitation encountered during the study was the difficulty in keeping seniors quiet during data collection. Since a wellness center already existed and seniors were accustomed to visiting with student nurses at a social level, it was difficult for them to refrain from talking during blood pressure measurement.

APPLICATION

Procedure guidelines for blood pressure measurement inconsistently address many factors that can affect blood pressure, in particular, the positioning of the feet (Anderson & Maloney, 1994). Clinical guidelines state that blood pressure should be measured while patients are seated in a chair with back supported and arms bared and supported at the heart level (Joint National Committee VI, 1997). According to the findings of this study and of Foster-Fitzpatrick et al. (1999), blood pressure readings may be artificially high if measured while an individual has a leg crossed at the knee. Even though results of this study were statistically significant, clinical significance may be limited. Systolic pressure changed only by 5.9 mmHg and diastolic changed by only 2.97 mmHg. Peters et al. (1999) did find that 18 out of 53 participants in their study were misclassified using blood pressure measurements taken with legs crossed and based on Joint National Committee VI risk classifications. Therefore, if a person's blood pressure measurement is already on the higher end of normal, even this small amount could affect that client's resulting treatment.

These findings can be immediately applied to all clinical settings where blood pressure measurement is a common function. Instructing patients to keep their feet flat on the floor during blood pressure measurement should be an important part of this procedure. Integration of this intervention into the procedure for taking blood pressure poses no untoward effects to patients. In fact, it should contribute to the quality of patient care, because accurate measurement and interpretation of blood pressure measurement is crucial in the assessment of a patient's health condition. It is also interesting to note that the biggest change in blood pressure readings with crossed legs was with the systolic pressure. Recent research supports the idea that systolic blood pressure is a better predictor of events (i.e., coronary heart disease, heart failure, stroke) than is the diastolic pressure in older persons (NIH Pub. No. 98-4080) (Joint National Committee, 1997). Schools of nursing should incorporate these findings into Fundamentals courses where basic skills such as blood pressure measurement are taught. Future research is needed to continue to build a body of evidence that supports both statistical and clinical significance. Replication of this study using larger samples and among more diverse populations and settings is recommended.

REFERENCES

Anderson, F. D., & Maloney, J. P. (1994). Taking blood pressure correctly: It's no off the cuff matter. *Nursing, 24*(11), 34–39.

Baker, R., & Ende J. (1995). Confounders of ausculatory blood pressure measurement. *Journal of General Internal Medicine, 10,* 223–230.

Bardwell, J. (1995). For good measure. *Nursing Times, 91*(27), 40–41.

Campbell, N., Hogan, D. B., & McKay, D. (1994). Pitfalls to avoid in the measurement of blood pressure in the elderly. *Canadian Journal of Public Health, 85* (Suppl. 2), S26–S29.

Campbell, N., & McKay, D. (1994). Accurate blood pressure why does it matter? *Canadian Medical Association Journal, 161*(3), 277–278.

Campbell, N., McKay, D., Chockalingam, A., & Fodor, J. (1994a). Errors in assessment of blood pressure measuring technique. *Canadian Journal of Public Health, 85*(Suppl. 2), S18–S21.

Campbell, N., McKay, D., Chockalingam, A., & Fodor, J. (1994b). Errors in assessment of blood pressure: Patient factors. *Canadian Journal of Public Health, 85*(Suppl. 2), S12–S17.

Campbell, N., McKay, D., Chockalingam, A., & Fodor, J. (1994c). Errors in assessment of blood pressure: Sphygmomanometers and blood pressure cuffs. *Canadian Journal of Public Health, 85*(S2), S22–S25.

Cohen, J. (1988). *Statistical power analysis for the behavioral sciences* (2nd ed.). Mahwah, NJ: Lawrence Erlbaum.

Cooper, K. M. (1992). Measuring blood pressure. The right way. *Nursing, 22*(4), 75.

Foster-Fitzpatrick, L., Ortiz, A., Siblano, H., Marcantonio, R., & Braun, L. T. (1999). The effect of crossed leg on blood pressure measurement. *Nursing Research, 48*(2), 105–107.

Frankel, D. (1999). How to measure blood pressure often forgotten. *Lancet, 353,* 1858.

Gillespie, A., & Curzio, J. (1998). Blood pressure measurement: Assessing staff knowledge. *Nursing Standard, 12,* 35–37.

Hill, M. N., & Grimm, C. M. (1991). How to take a precise blood pressure. *American Journal of Nursing, 91*(2), 38–42.

Hollander, J., & Singer, A. (1997). Blood pressure differences between arms. *Archives of Internal Medicine, 157*(7), 818.

Jamieson, M. J., Webster, J., Philips, S., Jeffers, T. A., Scott, A. K., Robb, O. J., et al. (1990). The measurement of blood pressure: Sitting or supine, once or twice? *Journal of Hypertension, 8,* 635–640.

Joint National Committee VI. (1997). *The sixth report of the Joint National Committee on prevention, detection, evaluation, and treatment of high blood pressure* (NIH Pub. No. 98-4080). USDHHS: Bethesda, MD.

Le Pailleur, C., Helft, G., Landais, P., Montgermont, P., Feder, J. M., Metzger, J. P., et al. (1998). The effects of talking, reading, and silence on the "white coat" phenomenon. *American Journal of Hypertension, 11,* 203–207.

Le Pailleur, C., Vacheron, A., Landais, P., Mounier-Vehier, C., Feder, J. M., Montgermont, P., et al. (1996). Talking effect and white coat phenomenon in hypertensive patients. *Behavioral Medicine, 22*(3), 114–122.

Moriera, L. B., Fuchs, F. D., Moraes, M., Bredemeier, M. B., & Duncan, B. B. (1998). Alcohol intake and blood pressure: The importance of time elapsed since last drink. *Journal of Hypertension, 16*(10), 1384–1386.

Netea, R. T., Smits, P., Lenders, J. W. M., & Thien, T. (1998). Does it matter whether blood pressure measurements are taken with subjects sitting or supine? *Journal of Hypertension, 16,* 262–268.

Netea, R. T., Smits, P., Lenders, J. W. M., & Thien, T. (1999). Arm position is important for blood pressure measurement. *Journal of Hypertension, 13*(2), 105–109.

Parati, G., Omboni, S., Staessen, J., Thijs, L., Fagard, R., Ulian, L., & Mancia, G. (1998). Limitations of the difference between clinic and daytime blood pressure as a surrogate measure of the 'white-coat' effect. *Journal of Hypertension, 16,* 23–29.

Perloff, D., Grim, C., Flack, J., Frohlich, E., Hill, M., McDonald, M., et al. (1993). Human blood pressure determination by syphygmomanometry. *Circulation, 88*(5, Pt. 1), 2460–2470.

Peters, G. L., Binder, S. K., & Campbell, N. R. (1999). The effect of crossing legs on blood pressure: A randomized single-blind cross-over study. *Blood Pressure Monitoring, 4,* 97–101.

Rudy, S. F. (1986). Take a reading on your blood pressure techniques. *Nursing, 16*(8), 46–49.

Sadowski, A. V., & Redeker, N. S. (1996). The hypertensive elder: A review for the primary care provider. *The Nurse Practitioner, 21*(5), 99–111.

Torrance, C. (1997). Practical procedures for nurses. *Nursing Times, 93,* 38.

Torrance, C., & Serginson, E. (1996). Student nurses' knowledge in relation to blood pressure measurement by sphygmomanometry and auscultation. *Nurse Education Today, 16,* 397–402.

van Lieshout, J. J., ten Harkel, A. D., & Wieling, W. (1992). Physical manoeuvres for combating orthostatic dizzieness in autonomic failure. *Lancet, 339,* 897–898.

Wieling, W., van Lieshout, J. J., & van Leeuwen, A. M. (1993). Physical manoeuvres that reduce postural hypotension in autonomic failure. *Clinical Autonomic Research, 3,* 57–65.

Rebecca Keele-Smith, Ph.D., A.P.R.N., B.C., is assistant professor in the Department of Nursing, New Mexico State University, Las Cruces.

CeCilia Price-Daniel, R.N., B.S.N., is a major in the Army Nurse Corps at the Army Medical Department Center and School, Fort Sam Houston, Texas. She is assigned to New Mexico State University as a full-time MSN student.

Evaluation of Individually Tailored Interventions on Exercise Adherence

REBECCA KEELE-SMITH
TERESA LEON

This study's purpose was to test the effects of a reversal theory–driven individualized exercise prescription on exercise consistency, weight, percentage body fat, and exercise motivation for a group of faculty, students, and staff at a southwestern university. Participants were randomly assigned to 5-week education plus monitoring or monitoring-only treatment groups. The hypothesis was that participants in the education plus monitoring group would have more consistent exercisers, higher exercise motivation scores, and greater overall weight loss and decrease in percentage of body fat than would those in the monitoring-only group. Consistent exercisers will score higher than inconsistent exercisers on exercise motivation scores. More participants were exercising at recommended levels in the education plus monitoring group than in the monitoring-only group after the study intervention. Consistent exercisers had significantly higher motivation scores than did inconsistent exercisers. Thus, individualized exercise prescriptions using reversal theory can be beneficial in promoting a consistent exercise program.

Keywords: exercise; motivation; physical activity

Consistent aerobic exercise results in many physiological and psychological benefits. Although the benefits of exercise are abundant, as little as 30% of the adult population in the United States remains committed to a regular exercise regimen (McAuley & Courneya, 1993). Motivation is an important determinant in predicting adherence; however, motives for exercising vary from individual to individual and have been difficult to measure consistently. Practitioners need to know these motives when designing exercise interventions. The Exercise Motivation Questionnaire (EMQ), developed to assess individual motives for exercising, shows promise in providing a foundation for developing

From "Evaluation of individually tailored interventions on exercise adherence," by R. Keele-Smith, & T. Leon, 2003, *Western Journal of Nursing Research 25*(6), 623–640. Copyright 2003 by Sage Publications. Reprinted with permission.

individualized exercise prescriptions that foster long-term adherence (Keele-Smith, 1999). The purpose of this study was to test the effects of individualized exercise prescriptions derived from the EMQ on exercise consistency, weight, percentage body fat, and exercise motivation for a group of faculty, students, and staff at a southwestern university in the United States.

FACTORS THAT AFFECT EXERCISE

Benefits

Physiological and psychological benefits of exercise justify the need to have physical fitness as a major health objective for the nation (U.S. Department of Health and Human Services, 2000). Research on regular aerobic exercise supports evidence of weight control, decreased resting heart rate and blood pressure, and increased cardiovascular endurance (Hooper & Veneziano, 1995; Paffenbarger et al., 1993). Regular exercise prevents and controls a variety of medical conditions and diseases such as obesity, diabetes mellitus, hypertension, and osteoporosis (Bouchard & Shephard, 1994; Helmrich, Ragland, & Leung, 1991; Lee, Paffenbarger, & Hsieh, 1991). Regular exercise also may help individuals by increasing energy levels and resistance to fatigue; increasing ability to cope with stress, anxiety, and depression; promoting relaxation; and improving sleep patterns and self-image (Whitmarsh, 1998). Exercising is expected to reduce morbidity, mortality, and health care costs while ultimately contributing to improved quality of life.

Barriers to Consistent Adherence

Although the benefits of exercise are well known, adherence rates are typically low. In fact, as much as 30% to 59% of the adult population in the United States has a sedentary lifestyle (McAuley & Courneya, 1993), and approximately 50% of individuals who do initiate an exercise program drop out within 3 to 6 months, well before any significant health benefits have been realized (Dishman, 1991; Robison & Rogers, 1994). Attrition continues until it levels off after 12 to 24 months (Martin & Dubbert, 1982).

Long-term adherence to an exercise program is a fundamental problem in the development of a healthy lifestyle. Reasons people stop exercising include injury, lack of direction, unrealistic goals, inability to slowly progress an exercise program, lack of professional guidance, lack of support, and unrealistic expectations with respect to weight loss (Sullivan, 1998). Dishman (1991) cited lack of motivation, discomforts during exercise, and smoking behavior as the most common personal characteristics directly related to decreased adherence and increased dropout from exercise programs.

Motivation and Exercise

Exercise motives can vary from person to person but may include health reasons, desire for fitness, weight control, personal appearance, socializing, wanting to feel better in general, increased energy, and goal commitment (Gillett, 1988; Shepard, 1985).

Assessing individual motives is important in understanding problems related to exercise adherence and for developing strategies and interventions to promote long-term adherence. Few instruments have been developed to assess individual motives for exercising and even fewer are based on theoretical models. One such instrument, the EMQ, was developed by Keele-Smith (2000).

Reversal theory, a theory of emotion, personality, and motivation (Apter, 1989), provided the foundation to develop the EMQ items.

REVERSAL THEORY AND EXERCISE

Reversal theory has been useful in explaining a variety of health-related behaviors such as gambling (Brown, 1991), relapse to smoking (O'Connell, Cook, Gerkovich, Potocky, & Swan, 1990; O'Connell, Potocky, Gerkovich, & Cook, 1993), weight cycling (Popkess-Vawter, Wendel, Schmoll, & O'Connell, 1998), sport and play (Apter, 1990; Kerr, 1991), and stress (Apter & Svebak, 1989). Also called the theory of psychological reversals, reversal theory holds that individuals are inherently inconsistent and that they reverse back and forth between opposing states of mind called meta-motivational states. The states are called meta-motivational because they influence how certain motivational variables such as arousal are experienced. Reversal theory espouses the following four pairs of opposing meta-motivational states: telic and paratelic, mastery and sympathy, negativistic and conformist, and autic and alloic (Apter, 1989). Meta-motivational states within a pair are mutually exclusive. One member of each of the pairs is said to be operative during all of waking life. Although one cannot be in both telic and paratelic states at the same time, one can, for example, be in paratelic, autic, mastery, and conformist states at the same time. The telic-paratelic and mastery-sympathy pairs, which appear to be the most relevant to exercise behavior, were used to provide structure and to develop items for the EMQ. Descriptions of each meta-motivational state can be found in **Table 1**.

Because people reverse back and forth between telic and paratelic states and between mastery and sympathy states, a single individual could experience exercise and preparations for engaging in exercise in several combinations of meta-motivational states: telic mastery, paratelic mastery, telic sympathy, and paratelic sympathy. To the extent that exercise meets the needs of various states, exercisers may recognize a variety of benefits or reasons for exercise that are consistent with one or more meta-motivational states. In addition, they may have developed strategies for maintaining exercise behavior that are consistent with particular states. These different reasons and strategies might operate both during and outside of exercise to influence the

Table 1   Descriptions of Meta-Motivational States Based on Reversal Theory

Telic	Exercise Intervention	Paratelic	Exercise Intervention
"End justifies the means." Goal is primary, and pleasure comes from movement toward the goal as well as attainment of the goal; serious-minded, future oriented.	Focus on goal setting, daily planning and/or weekly written schedule. Education could focus on exercise benefits such as weight management, feeling better, health reasons, decreased stress, long-term benefits, and so forth.	"Means justify the end." Activity is primary, and pleasure comes from the activity itself; playful, present oriented, spontaneous.	Encourage participation in exercise that they will truly enjoy, that requires minimal planning, and that is easily accessible. Encourage them to find an exercise partner that can support them by doing things such as helping them plan and get to the exercise activity.
Mastery		**Sympathy**	
Individuals see a situation in terms of a struggle, trial, test, or competition. They want to dominate or control.	Encourage participation in competitive exercise. Help set realistic expectations and selection of activities they can be successful in mastering.	Individual sees a situation in terms of cooperation, harmony, or nurturance and seeks to nurture or care for another or to be nurtured or cared for by another.	Encourage participation in something such as noncompetitive team sports or activities. Encourage them to find an exercise partner so they can help one another to maintain an exercise program. Encourage self-talk about how exercise is a way to take care of themselves and to make significant others proud of them.

Autocentric

Pleasure and displeasure derive primarily from what happens to the self.

Allocentric

Pleasure and displeasure derive primarily from what happens to others.

Negativistic

Pleasure comes from the need or desire to rebel against rules or conventions. Anger frequently occurs in this state.

Conformist

Pleasure comes from conforming to rules or conventions. There is an absence of rebelliousness.

continuation of an exercise regimen. For example, an individual may have paratelic reasons for doing the exercise but employ telic strategies for getting to the exercise session.

Although reversals are not totally under conscious control, there does seem to be a predisposition for an individual to be in a particular meta-motivational state in relation to certain situations or activities. For example, aerobic dance exercise tends to induce the paratelic state because of the circumstances surrounding the activity (e.g., lively music, stimulating exercises, or group effect). When a person engages in this activity, there is a greater probability of reversing to the paratelic state if telic or staying paratelic if that is the current state.

Exercise adherence research in the past has been characteristically atheoretical. Research with theoretical underpinnings has often produced findings with little connection to the theoretical explanations from which the measurements were developed (Dishman, 1982). The majority of studies had limited internal and external validity due to their nonexperimental designs. No research has been conducted using reversal theory to guide exercise interventions. This study will attempt to address this gap in the literature. Reversal theory offers a unique way to understand exercise adherence issues. For example, individuals who typically exercise in the paratelic state will have difficulty maintaining an exercise program if they pick an activity that they do not really enjoy. Example intervention strategies for each state can be found in Table 1.

HYPOTHESES

Participants in the education plus monitoring group will have a greater number of consistent exercisers and higher exercise motivation scores than will those in the monitoring-only group. Participants in the education plus monitoring group will have greater overall weight loss and decrease in percentage of body fat measurements than will those in the monitoring-only group. Consistent exercisers will score higher than will inconsistent exercisers on exercise motivation scores. The only treatment difference between the education plus monitoring group and the monitoring-only group is that the education plus monitoring group received an individualized exercise prescription based on participants exercise motivation scores, follow-up education, and reinforcement of their exercise prescription.

METHOD

Design

An experimental pretest-posttest design was used. Participants were randomly assigned through use of a random numbers table in an education plus monitoring or monitoring-only treatment group. Dependent variables included frequency and duration of exercise, weight, percentage body fat, and EMQ sub-scale scores measured at the beginning and the end of this 5-week study.

Consistency of exercise was measured by duration and frequency. Duration was measured as the current average time per exercise session across all types of exercise calculated in minutes. Frequency was the current total times per week for all types of current exercise. Participants were considered consistent exercisers if they were exercising at least 3 to 5 times per week for a minimum of 20 minutes each time. Participants were considered inconsistent exercisers if they were exercising less than this. Body fat percentage and weight were calculated using the TANITA Body Fat Monitor/Scale TBF-612 (TANITA, 1998). Exercise motivation was measured by calculating mean EMQ subscale scores.

Sample

Participants were faculty, staff, and students at a university in southwestern New Mexico. Participants included people who currently were having difficulty with their exercise programs or who wanted to initiate exercise programs. Difficulty was defined as not being able to maintain recommended levels of exercise consistently. Recommended levels of exercise included moderate to vigorous physical activity equivalent to at least sustained walking for a minimum of 20 to 30 minutes per session 3 to 5 times per week (American College of Sports Medicine, 1990; U.S. Department of Health and Human Services, 2000). Examples include walking, dancing, and yard work for moderate activity and running, aerobic dance, swimming, cycling, skating, skiing, or competitive group sports for vigorous activity.

Based on a power analysis using an alpha of .05, power of .80, and an effect size of .50, 63 participants per group were required. Participants were recruited by announcements made in college classes by researchers and instructors, by visiting exercise classes on campus, by word of mouth, and through the university's computer system hotline. A convenience sample of 149 adults was recruited. The attrition rate for this study was 3%, with 4 participants dropping out before the second set of measures were taken. There were no significant differences between those completing versus those dropping out of the study in gender, ethnicity, education, age, exercise status, marital status, or health status.

Of the 149 participants who participated in the study, 35 were male and 114 were female. Mean age was 31 (range = 18 to 59). A total of 75 participants were White (50.3%), 63 (42.3%) were Hispanic, 1 (0.7%) was African American, 4 (2.7%) were Asian, and 1 (0.7%) was Native American. Data were missing for 5 participants on ethnicity. This sample is fairly representative of this southern New Mexico county in which 40.7% of the population is White, 56% is Hispanic, 1.6% is African American, 0.9% is Asian, and 0.7%

is Native American (U.S. Department of Health, Public Health Division, 1997). The majority of the sample had at least some college education (67.1%). Most participants were married (53%), and many (49.7%) had at least one child. Few participants (10.7%) smoked. Most of the sample (75.8%) did not have a chronic disease. Of the 23.1% of the 34 participants who indicated a chronic disease, 10.7% had asthma as a chronic condition. Participants weighed an average of 164 (range = 98.5 to 289) pounds at the beginning of the study and 164 (range = 104 to 292.5) pounds at the end of the study. Mean percentage of body fat was 31.9 (range = 9% to 53%). At the beginning of the study, men weighed significantly more (mean = 180 vs. 159 pounds), $t(147) = -2.9$, $p = .003$, and had significantly less body fat than did women (mean = 20.5% vs. 35.4%), $t(147) = 8.7$, $p = < .001$).

Approval to conduct the study was obtained through the Human Participants Review Committee at the university where the principal investigator is a faculty member. Written informed consent indicated that participation was voluntary and that participants could withdraw from the study at anytime. Participants were instructed to consult with their health care provider regarding safety to participate if they had a health risk factor that could affect their ability to exercise (e.g., hypertension, diabetes, heart disease, or obesity).

Measures

The TANITA Body Fat Monitor/Scale TBF-612 was used to measure weight and body fat. The TANITA scale uses the bioelectrical impedance analysis technique. In this method, a low level electrical signal is passed through the body. It is difficult for a signal to flow through fat in the human body but easy to flow through moisture in the muscle and other body tissues. High correlations (within 3% to 5%) with standard methods of fat percentage measurement such as dual-energy x-ray absorptiometry and hydrodensitometry (underwater weighing) have been reported (TANITA, 1998). Weight was measured to the nearest 0.5 pound, and fat was measured to the nearest 1%. Measurements were taken at the same time of day, and participants were encouraged to wear similar clothing for both pre- and postweight and fat measurements.

Participants were asked to complete the 55-item EMQ. Choices ranged from *strongly agree* to *strongly disagree* on the 1 to 4 Likert-type scale. Developed from reversal theory constructs, the EMQ contains four subscales: Experience of Exercise, Prevention of Negative Feelings, Planning/Commitment, and Social Support. The Experience of Exercise subscale contains paratelic-mastery motives, the Prevention of Negative Feelings subscale contains telic-mastery motives, the Planning/Commitment subscale contains telic motives, and the Social Support subscale contains sympathy motives. For example, "Exercise is an enjoyable experience for me" is an item from the Experience of Exercise subscale. The subscale Prevention of Negative Feelings includes items such as "I feel guilty when I'm not able to exercise because I know it is one way that I can take care of myself." The Planning/Commitment subscale contains items that have to do with getting to the exercise session, such as "I plan my day so that I can exercise." The Social Support subscale includes items such as "I exercise because my spouse/friend wants me to." Initial development of the EMQ resulted in subscale reliabilities all within an acceptable range as demonstrated by the following alphas: Experience of Exercise subscale = .95, Prevention of Negative Feelings subscale = .90, Planning/Commitment subscale = .87, and Social Support subscale = .75 (Keele-Smith, 2000). Cronbach's alpha for the EMQ subscales for this study were also acceptable and ranged from .70 to .94 in the first administration at the beginning of the study and from .73 to .95 in the second administration at the completion of the study.

Initial evidence of convergent and discriminant validity has been shown by predicted significant positive relationships between the EMQ and Markland and Hardy's (1993) Exercise Motivation Inventory (Keele-Smith, 2000). See **Table 2** for specific subscale correlations.

A weekly exercise questionnaire was also completed by interview with the participants to ascertain a summary of their exercise activity for the week. For example, participants in the monitoring-only group were asked about the type, duration, and frequency of their exercise activity for the week and about any barriers that interfered with their ability to exercise. Participants in the education plus monitoring group were asked similar questions, plus time was spent discussing their individualized exercise plans and continued strategies for maintaining their programs including any educational needs that were identified.

Procedures

Both groups filled out the EMQ and the demographic questionnaire at the beginning of the study and again at the end of the study. Weight and fat measurements also were taken at the beginning and the end of the study. Graduate nursing and public health students enrolled in a graduate research class performed the measurements. Training sessions were conducted for the research students. Students had to perform the procedure correctly a minimum of two times without error before continuing. Weekly contacts for 5 weeks were made for all participants.

Participants in the education plus monitoring group initially received a brochure that highlighted general information about exercise. Information included recommendations for exercise activity, benefits of exercise, potential barriers to exercising (anticipatory guidance), and examples of interventions or strategies to use to increase adherence. Participants in the education plus monitoring group had their EMQ scores analyzed during the first week of the study.

Table 2   Convergent and Discriminant Validity of the Exercise Motivation Questionnaire (EMQ)

| | EMQ Subscale | | | |
Exercise Motivation Inventory Subscale	Experience of Exercise	Social Support	Prevention of Negative Feelings	Planning/ Commitment
Revitalization	.59[a]			
Enjoyment	.70[a]	−.003[b]		.04[b]
Challenge	.66[a]	.13[b]		
Competition	.45[a]			
Strength	.55[a]			
Nimbleness	.31[a]			
Social Recognition		.32[a]		
Affiliation		.33[a]		
Stress Management		−.06[b]	.24[a]	.02[b]
Ill-Health Avoidance	.17[b]		.23[a]	
Positive Health		−.06[b]	.41[a]	
Weight Management	.11[b]	.09[b]	.39[a]	
Appearance		.08[b]	.52[a]	
Health Pressures	.02[b]			

a. Significant positive relationships.
b. Minimal or negative relationships.

An individualized written exercise prescription was developed by the principal investigator based on how the participants endorsed motives for exercising on the EMQ. The prescription included suggestions on the type, frequency, and duration of exercise and strategies for increasing compliance. For example, a participant who had high scores on the Experience of Exercise and Prevention of Negative feelings subscales but low scores on the Social Support and Planning/Commitment subscales was given strategies such as learning time management skills and finding friends and/or family willing to help. Goal setting, prioritizing, making a written schedule, asking a friend or family member to baby-sit, making reminder phone calls, or actually exercising with another person are specific examples of interventions that were suggested. Along with the written exercise prescription, research assistants provided individualized, one-on-one weekly education sessions that lasted approximately 30 to 45 minutes to help participants follow the prescription. Participants were also asked to describe type, frequency, and duration of exercise activity for each of the 5 weeks.

Participants in the monitoring-only group received weekly contacts by telephone. Questions focused on participants' exercise activities for the week. Strategies that seemed to help them exercise and barriers to exercise activity were assessed. They were also asked to describe current type, frequency, and duration of exercise for the week the same as was the education plus monitoring group. They received the initial brochure that the other intervention group got during the first week, but they did not receive an individualized exercise prescription, follow-up education, or any advice on how to improve their exercise activities.

Data Analysis

Independent sample t tests will be conducted on between-group differences, and paired sample t tests will be performed on within-group differences between weight, percentage body fat, and EMQ subscale scores. To examine differences in exercise motivation subscale scores between participants who were consistently exercising and participants who were not, independent sample t tests will be completed. For categorical data such as age, gender, ethnicity, and education, the cross-tabs procedure will be used to detect any significant differences between groups on EMQ subscale scores and consistency of exercise.

FINDINGS

Differences Between Groups

No significant differences were found between groups at the beginning and end of the study on age, gender, ethnicity, education, marital status, smoking, presence of chronic illnesses, weight, percentage of body fat, and EMQ subscale scores. Significant differences were found between consistency of exercise and group membership at the end of the study, as demonstrated by the cross-tabs procedure (Cramer's V = .174, p = .04). At pretest, no significant differences in consistency of exercise were found between treatment groups. Out of 137 participants without missing data (N = 149), only 27 in the education plus monitoring and 31 in the monitoring-only group were consistently exercising at pretest. Out of 144 participants without missing data (N = 149), significantly more participants were exercising at recommended levels in the education plus monitoring group (n = 37) than in the monitoring-only group

($n = 23$) after the study intervention. At the end of the study, there were 10 more participants consistently exercising in the education plus monitoring group (37 vs. 27) and 8 more participants not consistently exercising in the monitoring-only group (31 vs. 23).

Differences Within Groups

To test for within-group differences between weight, percentage body fat, and EMQ subscale scores, paired sample t tests were performed. There were no significant pretest to posttest differences found on weight or percentage of body fat, but weight and percentage of body fat dropped slightly for both groups. An average of 1.3 and 0.75 pounds were lost from beginning to end for the education plus monitoring and monitoring-only groups, respectively. On average, participants in the education plus monitoring group lost 0.5% body fat and the monitoring only group actually gained 0.3% body fat. Both the education plus monitoring and the monitoring-only groups showed significant improvement in Planning/Commitment subscale scores, 15.1 ± 4.1 to 16.3 ± 4.3, $t(72) = -2.4$, $p = .02$; 15.2 ± 4.3 to 16.6 ± 4.1, $t(71) = -2.8$, $p = .01$. The education plus monitoring group also showed significant improvement in social support scores, 9.9 ± 3.1 to 10.7 ± 3.1, $t(71) = -4.55$, $p = .03$, whereas the monitoring only group showed significant improvement in experience of exercise scores, 64.1 ± 13.9 to 67 ± 15, $t(67) = -2.29$, $p = .03$.

Exercise Motivation and EMQ Scores

To examine differences in exercise motivation subscale scores between participants who were consistently exercising and participants who were not, independent sample t tests were performed. Consistent exercisers had significantly higher experience of exercise, prevention of negative feelings, and planning/commitment scores than did inconsistent exercisers both at the beginning of the study and at completion. See **Table 3** for specific findings of these analyses.

Further Analyses

Because significant differences were found between exercise status and group membership at the end of the study, further analyses were performed examining participants' exercise status at the beginning and at the end of the study. Participants who were exercising at the beginning of the study ($n = 58$) endorsed more than one type of exercise and averaged three times per week (ranging from 1 to 12 times per week) across all types of current exercise. Average duration per session was 45 minutes, and the mean length of time they had been exercising consistently was 3.9 years. Participants who were not currently exercising ($n = 79$) also endorsed most frequently more than one type

Table 3 **Significant Results of Independent Sample *t* Tests Comparing Consistent Exercisers With Inconsistent Exercisers on Exercise Motivation Questionnaire Subscale Score**

	t Test			Consistent Exercisers		Inconsistent Exercisers	
	n	t	p	M	SD	M	SD
Start of study							
Experience of Exercise	137	3.64	< .0001	69.72	12.94	61.59	12.88
Prevention of Negative Feelings	137	2.89	.005	52.95	8.59	48.17	10.24
Planning/Commitment	137	4.83	< .0001	17.26	3.82	14.04	3.89
Social Support	137	0.68	.49	10.12	3.06	9.76	3.10
End of study							
Experience of Exercise	140	2.84	.005	70.60	12.24	64.33	13.33
Prevention of Negative Feelings	141	2.55	.012	53.00	8.72	48.92	9.75
Planning/Commitment	142	4.79	< .0001	18.25	3.58	15.12	4.01
Social Support	141	0.30	.76	10.71	3.22	10.55	3.11

NOTE: Sample sizes are different because of missing data.
Total sample size = 149.

of exercise. Mean length of time since exercising consistently was 3.2 years, and mean length of time consistently exercising before quitting was 1.7 years. The most frequently reported form of exercise for both groups was walking. As a group, participants at the end of the study who were unable to maintain a consistent exercise program versus those who did tended to be female (80% vs. 69%), to smoke (13% vs. 5%), and to be more culturally diverse (51% vs. 46%) than were consistent exercisers.

DISCUSSION

The primary purpose of this study was to test the effects of individualized exercise interventions on exercise consistency, exercise motivation scores, weight, and percentage body fat for a group of faculty, students, and staff at a southwestern New Mexico university. Overall, participants were very healthy, young, well-educated, and ethnically representative of the geographical area.

Demographic findings of this study are similar to what Buckworth (2000) summarized in a meta-analysis as consistent correlates of exercise and physical activity. Buckworth identified demographic characteristics such as gender, age, ethnicity, education, income, and occupation as important determinants of exercise and physical activity. Women are more likely to be inactive than men. Significantly more men than women report vigorous physical activity. Participation in physical activity tends to decrease as individuals get older. Whites are more physically active than are other racial/ethnic groups regardless of age. Other studies have found that declines in physical activity in adults over time are associated with lower education, low income, blue-collar occupations, social isolation, marital status (unmarried), smoking, and perceived poor health status. In general, similar findings were found in this study. As a group, participants who were unable to maintain a consistent exercise program versus those who did tended to be of an ethnic minority, to be female, and to smoke.

One of the most important findings of this study was that participants in the group that received the individually tailored exercise prescription had significantly more consistent exercisers and fewer inconsistent exercisers than did those who only received monitoring. These posttest differences may result from both an increase in consistent exercisers in the education plus monitoring group and a decrease of consistent exercisers in the monitoring-only group. Findings suggest that this particular intervention helps people to not only increase their consistency in exercise but also helps maintain a consistent program once established. This supports the underlying theoretical concepts from reversal theory. Motives behind individuals' behavior can vary, and knowledge of these motives is important in developing strategies to promote compliance with health promotion activities such as exercise. Implementing an individualized exercise prescription incorporating these motives demonstrated that compliance could be improved and/or maintained during this study.

Another important finding is that the EMQ tended to discriminate between consistent and inconsistent exercisers within this study. Scores on the EMQ may be helpful in predicting future adherence to an exercise program. Except for the Social Support subscale, consistent exercisers scored significantly higher than did inconsistent exercisers on the EMQ subscales at both the beginning and the end of the study. Although scores on the Social Support subscale were not significantly different between consistent and inconsistent exercisers, consistent exercisers did score higher on average than did inconsistent exercisers. One reason that the social support may have not discriminated as well as the other subscales is it had the weakest measure of internal consistency (.75) and contained the smallest number of items (6). More work is needed to improve this subscale's reliability.

One of the major strengths of this study was the ability to maintain a minimal attrition rate (3%). Weekly contacts, reminders of appointments, and making a concerted effort to work around participants' schedules contributed to the low attrition.

No significant differences were found between the education plus monitoring and monitoring-only groups on weight loss or percentage body fat measurement at the end of the study. One of the main limitations of this study was that it was only 5 weeks long, perhaps not long enough to see much change especially with weight and body fat measurement. This study was done as part of a semester-long graduate nursing research class and was limited to 5 weeks of actual data collection. Due to these time limitations, exercise motivation and compliance alone may have been more realistic measures of the usefulness of the EMQ. Resulting trends, however, were promising even after this short time period. Another limitation was that data were collected by self-report. Actual observation or other measures of validation in future work would strengthen study design. Another area where the study design could be strengthened in the future is in the sampling criteria. Several participants ($n = 69$) in this study were already exercising consistently. They were included in this study because they wanted to improve their consistency over time. Although they were consistently exercising at the time of the study, all verbalized recent difficulties in maintaining an exercise program at the recommended levels for any length of time. To maximize differences between groups, sampling criteria could be focused on individuals wanting to start an exercise program or only exercising sporadically.

As demonstrated by this study, intervention strategies to promote consistent exercise can be individually tailored according to how one scores on the EMQ. Strategies for people with high scores on the Experience of Exercise subscale might include finding an exercise activity that is fun and challenging. Examples could include use of music, socializing and group cohesion, positive sensations of the exercise experience, pleasurable feelings associated with increased energy and fitness, mastering the exercise, competition with one's self or with others, and promotion of a sense of accomplishment and progress. For people with high scores on the Prevention of Negative Feelings subscale, interventions that emphasize self-talk about how exercising will prevent them from feeling tired, depressed, or anxious could be included. An exercise activity that is less intense and challenging might also be more appropriate with these individuals.

Few instruments with adequate validity and reliability have been developed to assess motives for exercising, and even fewer are based on theoretical constructs. Most research in the past has been at the nonexperimental level. This study's purpose was to improve on all of these weaknesses. Based on reversal theory, the EMQ demonstrated good validity and reliability in this group of participants. Consistent exercisers scored significantly higher on three of the four EMQ subscales. Participants that received the individualized prescription maintained or improved their exercise compliance.

The benefits of exercise are well known. Research supports that people who maintain a wellness-oriented lifestyle are happier, more productive, and tend to use less acute care medical services. Consistent exercise is now seen as an integral piece of a wellness lifestyle. Participation in exercise can be expected to reduce morbidity, mortality, and health care costs and ultimately to improve quality of life. Even so, exercise adherence rates are low and dropouts are common. To improve adherence, it is imperative to develop and test strategies such as the individualized exercise prescription tested here.

NOTE

1. We would like to thank the following students from New Mexico State University for their help in designing this study, recruiting participants, and collecting data: M.S.N. students Karen Lee, Diane Turner, Linda Shaberg, Kerry Harris, Shannon Rodriguez, Lisa Taylor, Veronica Malone, Chris King, Myong O'Donnell, Sally Perry, Maj-Liz Downey, and Debbie Cates; and M.P.H. students Jim Farmer, Danial Khan, Casilda Provencio, Becky Elliot, and Josefina Ramirez.

REFERENCES

American College of Sports Medicine. (1990). The recommended quantity and quality of exercise for developing and maintaining cardiorespiratory and muscular fitness in healthy adults. *Medicine and Science in Sports and Exercise, 22*(2), 265–274.

Apter, M. J. (1989). *Reversal theory: Motivation, emotion, and personality.* Boston, MA: Routledge Kegan Paul.

Apter, M. J. (1990). Sport and mental health: A new psychological perspective. In G. P. H. Hermans & W. L. Mosterd (Eds.), *Sports, medicine, and health* (pp. 47–56). New York, NY: Elsevier-North Holland.

Apter, M. J., & Svebak, S. (1989). Stress from the reversal theory perspective. In C. D. Spielberger & J. Strelau (Eds.), *Stress and anxiety* (pp. 12–15). New York, NY: Hemisphere/ McGraw.

Bouchard, C., & Shephard, R. (1994). Consensus statement. In C. Bouchard, R. Shephard, & T. Stephens (Eds.), *Physical activity, fitness, and health: International proceedings and consensus statement.* Champaign, IL: Human Kinetics.

Brown, R. I. F. (1991). Gambling, gaming and other addictive play. In J. H. Kerr & M. J. Apter (Eds.), *Adult play: A reversal theory approach* (pp. 101–118). Amsterdam, The Netherlands: Swets and Zeitlinger.

Buckworth, J. (2000). Exercise determinants and interventions. *International Journal of Sport Psychology, 31,* 305–320.

Dishman, R. (1982). Compliance/adherence in health related exercise. *Health Psychology, 3,* 237–267.

Dishman, R. (1991). Increasing and maintaining exercise and physical activity. *Behavior Therapy, 22,* 345–377.

Gillett, P. (1988). Self-reported factors influencing exercise adherence in overweight women. *Nursing Research, 37,* 25–28.

Helmrich, S., Ragland, D., & Leung, R. (1991). Physical activity and reduced occurrence of non-insulin-dependent diabetes mellitus. *New England Journal of Medicine, 325,* 147–152.

Hooper, J., & Veneziano, L. (1995). Distinguishing starters from nonstarters in an employee physical activity incentive program. *Health Education Quarterly, 22,* 49–58.

Keele-Smith, R. (1999). *Reversal theory and motivational factors for exercising* (UMI No. 9991623). Lawrence, KS: University of Kansas.

Kerr, J. H. (1991). Arousal-seeking in risk sports participants. *Personality and Individual Differences, 12,* 613–616.

Lee, I., Paffenbarger, R., & Hsieh, C. (1991). Physical activity and risk of developing colorectal cancer among college alumni. *Journal National Cancer Institute, 83,* 1324–1329.

Markland, D., & Hardy, L. (1993). The exercise motivations inventory: Preliminary development and validity of a measure of individuals' reasons for participation in regular physical exercise. *Personality and Individual Differences, 15,* 289–296.

Martin, J., & Dubbert, P. (1982). Exercise applications and promotions in behavioral medicine: Current status and future directions. *Journal of Consulting and Clinical Psychology, 50,* 1004–1017.

McAuley, E., & Courneya, K. (1993). Adherence to exercise and physical activity as health-promoting behaviors: Attitudinal and self-efficacy influences. *Applied and Preventative Psychology, 2,* 65–77.

O'Connell, K. A., Cook, M. R., Gerkovich, M. M., Potocky, M., & Swan, G. E. (1990). Reversal theory and smoking: A state-based approached to ex-smokers' highly tempting situations. *Journal of Consulting and Clinical Psychology, 58,* 489–494.

O'Connell, K. A., Potocky, M., Gerkovich, M. M., & Cook, M. R. (1993). A reversal theory approach for categorizing strategies used to cope with temptations to smoke. In J. H. Kerr, S. Murgatroyd, & J. J. Apter (Eds.), *Advances in reversal theory* (pp. 225–234). Amsterdam, The Netherlands: Swets and Zeitlinger.

Paffenbarger, R. S., Hyder, R. T., Wind, A. L., Lee, I., Jung, D. L., & Kampter, J. B. (1993). The association of changes in physical activity level and other lifestyle characteristics with mortality among men. *New England Journal of Medicine, 328,* 538–545.

Popkess-Vawter, S., Wendel, S., Schmoll, S., & O'Connell, K. (1998). Overeating, reversal theory, and weight cycling. *Western Journal of Nursing Research, 20,* 67–83.

Robison, J., & Rogers, M. (1994). Adherence to exercise programs. *Sports Medicine, 17,* 39–52.

Shepard, R. (1985). Factors influencing the exercise behavior of patients. *Sports Medicine, 2,* 348–365.

Sullivan, D. (1998). Beat the odds! *Joe Weider's Shape, 17,* 126–129.

TANITA. (1998). TBF-612 *Body Fat Monitor/Scale instruction manual* [Brochure]. Arlington Heights, IL: TANITA Corporation.

U.S. Department of Health and Human Services. (2000). *Healthy people 2010: National health promotion and disease prevention objectives.* (DHHS Publication No. 91-30212). Washington, DC: Author.

U.S. Department of Health, Public Health Division. (1997). *1997 New Mexico selected health statistics annual report.* Santa Fe, NM: State Center for Health Statistics.

Whitmarsh, B. (1998). Psych fitness. *Joe Weider's Muscle and Fitness, 59,* 124–127.

Rebecca Keele-Smith, Ph.D., APRN, BC, Assistant Professor, New Mexico State University, Department of Nursing

Teresa Leon, BCH, R.N., M.S.N. Graduate Student, New Mexico State University, Department of Nursing.

Transforming the Death Sentence: Elements of Hope in Women With Advanced Ovarian Cancer

ANNE M. REB, PhD, NP

Purpose/Objectives: To describe the experience of hope in women with advanced ovarian cancer.

Research Approach: Grounded theory methodology with interviews.

Setting: Oncology clinics in the northeastern United States.

Participants: 20 women aged 42–73 who had completed initial chemotherapy and had no evidence of recurrence.

Methodologic Approach: A personal data form and focused interview guide supported data collection. The core variable and related themes were identified using the constant comparative process. Demographic and treatment information was analyzed using descriptive statistics.

Main Research Variables: The process of hope in women with advanced ovarian cancer.

Findings: Facing the death sentence emerged as the main concern. The core variable in dealing with the concern was transforming the death threat. The three phases of the trajectory were shock (reverberating from the impact), aftershock (grasping reality), and rebuilding (living the new paradigm). Health-care provider communication and spirituality influenced women's abilities to transform the death sentence. Support and perceived control emerged as key dimensions of the core variable.

From "Transforming the death sentence: Elements of hope in women with advanced ovarian cancer," by A. M. Reb, 2007, *Oncology Nursing Forum, 34*(6), E70–E81. Copyright 2007 by the Oncology Nursing Society. Reprinted with permission.

Conclusions: Women experience significant distress and trauma symptoms associated with a diagnosis of ovarian cancer. Hope was linked closely to the core variable and was necessary for finding meaning in the experience. Women with high support and perceived control seemed most hopeful and able to transform the death sentence.

Interpretations: Evidence-based interventions and strategies are needed to foster improved provider communication, symptom management, and peer support for women facing ovarian cancer. Future nursing research should focus on strategies that enhance support, perceived control, hope, and spirituality.

KEY POINTS

- Life-threatening illnesses such as ovarian cancer are associated with loss of control.
- Shifting expectations, focusing on realistic goals, and finding meaning in the cancer experience enhanced women's sense of control.
- Provider communication and spirituality provided a context that influenced women's abilities to transform the death sentence.
- Perceived support and control emerged as key dimensions of the core variable that influenced women's hopes.

Approximately two-thirds of women diagnosed with ovarian cancer have advanced disease because the disease is difficult to diagnose in its early stages. Survivorship issues are becoming increasingly important as women live longer and treatment and supportive care for ovarian cancer improve (Christopher, 2006; Ferrell, Virani, Smith, & Juarez, 2003; Payne, 2006). Women with ovarian cancer have identified significant quality-of-life (QOL) concerns, including threats to physical, social, spiritual, and functional well-being (Cella, 1994; Ersek, Ferrell, Dow, & Melancon, 1997; Ferrell et al., 2005). Newly diagnosed women also experience significant levels of trauma symptoms, such as intrusive thoughts and avoidance behaviors (Posluszny, 2001), including a sustained trauma characterized by "living in the face of death" (Thompson, 2005, p. 72). Some prominent themes in recent studies include hope and finding meaning (Bowes, Tamlyn, & Butler, 2002; Sivesind & Baile, 1997). Hope is a dynamic process believed to change over time (Cutcliffe, 1996; Farran, Herth, & Popovich, 1995; Herth, 1990; Nowotny, 1989) and is "characterized by a confident yet uncertain expectation of achieving a future good, which to the hoping person is realistically possible and personally significant" (Dufault & Martocchio, 1985, p. 380). Although a cancer diagnosis may threaten one's hope (Rustoen & Hanestad, 1998), maintaining hope can provide meaning and direction (Bowes et al.; Post-White et al., 1996) and is associated with improved coping and QOL (Ballard, Green, McCaa, & Logsdon, 1997; Chi, 2007; Herth & Cutcliffe, 2002a; Post-White et al.; Rustoen, 1995). Hope has been explored in diverse contexts, including patients with advanced cancer or HIV, palliative care, and terminal illness (Buckley & Herth, 2004; Herth & Cutcliffe, 2002a). Limited research has addressed hope in women with ovarian cancer, and further research is needed to address hope and QOL concerns associated with long-term treatment (Ferrell et al., 2005; McCorkle, Pasacreta, & Tang, 2003). The purpose of this study was to describe the experience of hope in women with advanced ovarian cancer. The study used grounded theory methodology with an interview approach.

CONCEPTUAL ORIENTATION

With the grounded theory method, a comprehensive literature review is not done initially so that the substantive theory emerges from the participant data. When the theory is sufficiently developed, relevant literature is integrated as it relates to the emerging theory (Glaser, 1978; Stern, 1980; Wolcott, 2002). The conceptual orientation underlying this research was based on symbolic interactionism and constructivist paradigms. Symbolic interactionism focuses on meaning that arises through social interaction and is modified through interpretations that influence actions (Annells, 1996; Blumer, 1969). A constructivist approach recognizes the interactive nature of data collection and analysis (Guba & Lincoln, 1989; Lincoln & Guba, 2000) and emphasizes mutually created constructions that allow the data to guide the investigator (Glaser, 1978; Glaser & Strauss, 1967).

METHODS

Design

The present study used a modified version of grounded theory based on Glaser and Strauss's (1967) classic work and Glaser's (1978, 1992) updates. The method is appropriate for the topic because grounded theory is process oriented and seeks to discover theoretical explanations when little information is available on a topic.

Participants and Setting

Purposive sampling was used to identify women with a diagnosis of stage III or IV ovarian cancer who had completed an initial course of chemotherapy and had no evidence of recurrence at the time of interview. Women within five years of diagnosis and with no other life-threatening comorbidities were eligible. Participants were recruited from oncology clinics at two community-based hospitals, two large teaching hospitals, and a private group hematology and oncology practice in the northeastern United States. Permission was obtained from the respective institutional review boards and a university's committee on protection of human subjects. Interviews were conducted at participants' or close family members' homes, workplaces, treatment facilities, and a local restaurant.

Instruments

Two instruments were used to support data collection: a **personal data form** and a **focused interview guide**. The personal data form included demographic, illness, and treatment-related questions. The interview guide (see **Figure 1**) was developed by the investigator and included open-ended questions about women's experiences of hope. Questions were based on a preliminary literature review of the concept of hope with input from clinical nurse experts and doctorally prepared nurses with expertise in grounded theory method. New interview questions were added to address emerging themes as guided by the ongoing analysis (Hutchinson & Wilson, 2001). Participants were asked to tell about their experiences of diagnosis and treatment at the start of the interviews.

Procedures

Most referrals came from clinic nurses and a few from the medical or surgical oncologists. Those providers performed initial screening and obtained

---

Figure 1   Initial Interview Guide

1. What does the word "hope" mean to you personally?
2. Tell me about your experience of hope before being diagnosed with cancer.
3. Can you identify any experiences, people, or situations that have influenced your hope since your diagnosis with cancer?
4. Tell me about your experience of hope since being diagnosed with ovarian cancer.
5. Describe any changes in your hope since your diagnosis.
6. What gives you the most hope at the present time?
7. Some women have identified concerns related to their diagnosis or situations that threaten their hope. Can you describe any experiences that have made you feel less hopeful?
8. Is there anything else you would like to add about your experience of hope?

permission to relay contact information. Informed consent was obtained, and participants were given a copy of the personal data form to complete prior to the interview meeting. Each participant identified a pseudonym used to label tapes and transcriptions. Interviews lasted one and a half to two hours and were taped and transcribed verbatim by experienced transcriptionists. Data were collected until saturation or when no new themes emerged related to the categories (Hutchinson & Wilson, 2001). Saturation of the categories occurred after completion of about 17 interviews; however, three additional interviews were analyzed to ensure saturation and include all enrolled participants.

Data Analysis

Data were analyzed concurrently using the constant comparative process to guide subsequent data collection (Glaser, 1978; Glaser & Strauss, 1967). Initial analysis consisted of reading the entire transcript followed by line-by-line coding to identify all key concepts. Ethnograph 5.08 (Qualis Research Associates) software was used to record memos and label key text segments with succinct codes. Similar incidents were combined into categories with the goal of accounting for the core variable that helped participants deal with their main concerns. The core variable is the central theme that relates to the many categories and accounts for most of the variation in the data. The variable was classified as a basic social process because it represented a trajectory of stages occurring over time. Theoretical coding was employed to conceptualize how the substantive codes relate to each other. In addition, methodologic and theoretical memos were written to focus the categories and increase the conceptual level of the data. Trustworthiness of the data was addressed through close adherence to the method and included classic techniques such as credibility, transferability, dependability, and confirmability (Lincoln & Guba, 1985, 2000). Credibility was addressed, in part, through analysis of negative cases to ensure fit of the data with the emerging theory (Lincoln & Guba, 1985; Patton, 1990; Sandelowski, 1986). Nurses with expertise in grounded theory method audited several transcripts and examined process issues and data interpretations. In addition, one participant commented on the findings during the final stages of analysis.

RESULTS

Participant Characteristics

Twenty women met the eligibility criteria and agreed to participate (see **Table 1**). Most women were diagnosed with stage III epithelial ovarian cancer; most were Caucasian, post-menopausal, and married with children. The mean age was 58 years (range = 42–73 years). Four women had children age 12 or younger. Fifty percent held a college degree or higher.

Table 1   Participant Characteristics

Characteristic	$\overline{X}$	Range
Age (years)	58	42–73
Months since initial diagnosis	15	7–49

Characteristic	n	%
Diagnosis		
Epithelial ovarian cancer	18	90
Primary peritoneal cancer	2	10
Stage		
III	15	75
IV	5	25
Race		
African American	3	15
Caucasian	17	85
Income ($) (N = 14)		
< 20,000	2	14
20,000–40,000	2	14
41,000–60,000	5	36
61,000–80,000	3	21
> 81,000	2	14
Education		
High school graduate	4	20
Some college	6	30
College degree	5	25
Some postgraduate	1	5
Master's degree	4	20
Employment status		
Employed	7	35
Unemployed	1	5
Retired	10	50
Medical leave	2	10
Religious preference[a]		
Christian	3	15
Catholic	7	35
Protestant	9	45
Jewish	1	5
Marital status		
Single	1	5
Married	13	65
Divorced	2	10
Widowed	4	20

N = 20

[a] Religious preference was self-reported by participants.

Note. Because of rounding, not all percentages total 100.

Overview: Facing the Death Threat

Most women had been healthy prior to diagnosis and their lives were greatly changed on receiving the news. Women experienced significant losses and changes as they dealt with the physical and psychological impact and reported challenges such as living with ongoing uncertainty and fears of recurrence and death. One participant described the experience as "rebuilding from ground zero." Acknowledging the reality of a poor prognosis occurred over time as women dealt with their main concern, facing the death threat. The basic social process, or core variable, that helped women deal with the concern was transforming the death sentence. Although individual responses varied, the process involved three major phases: shock (reverberating from the impact), aftershock (grasping reality), and rebuilding (living the new paradigm) (see **Figure 2**). Women's abilities to move through the phases were influenced by perceived levels of support and control, which emerged as key dimensions of the core variable.

Hope and the core variable: Although hope did not emerge as the participants' main concern, it was closely linked to the core variable. Women described hope as a feeling that changed over time and associated it with the ability to return to normal, participate in meaningful activities, and survive the disease. Most women expressed that hope needed reinforcement (Penrod & Morse, 1997) and described strategies and situations that supported and threatened their hope. Hope played a key role as a condition and a consequence of transforming the death sentence and was necessary for finding meaning (Bowes et al., 2002). Hope as a condition was dynamic and associated with certain recurring contextual themes related to the core variable.

Figure 2   Phases: Transforming the Death Sentence

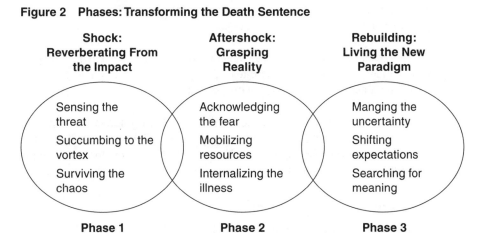

Shock: Reverberating From the Impact	Aftershock: Grasping Reality	Rebuilding: Living the New Paradigm
Sensing the threat	Acknowledging the fear	Manging the uncertainty
Succumbing to the vortex	Mobilizing resources	Shifting expectations
Surviving the chaos	Internalizing the illness	Searching for meaning
Phase 1	**Phase 2**	**Phase 3**

Healthcare provider communication and spirituality: Contextual themes, including healthcare provider communication and spirituality, recurred through-out the phases and influenced women's abilities to transform the death sentence. Because ovarian cancer is less common than other cancers, many women did not immediately understand the implications and relied on their providers for cues for interpreting the illness. Communication was perceived as a process over time as women tried to understand the meaning of the illness. Women were sensitive to providers' communications and almost hypervigilant in monitoring their responses. Several women relied on their providers' assessment, and most felt more hopeful as a result. Women valued communications that were honest yet optimistic and were encouraged on hearing positive information.

> I think when I met Dr. M, to me that was probably when my hope changed when he said, "No, this doesn't have to be a death sentence. We treat this as more like a chronic illness and we follow it that way." That gave me a lot of hope when he just said that to me.

Alternatively, women who experienced negative communications felt more anx-ious and less hopeful.

> I guess at one point towards the end, it was made to sound like I could just expect a recurrence and I was very surprised at that. . . . So, I think that was probably the most disconcerting thing I could have heard. . . . I said, "Well I'm just gonna set that aside. . . . Try to keep that out of your mind too much, because you don't want to . . . deal with it."

Several women relied on spirituality and their relationship with God or a higher power as a source of hope and comfort. Although women were fright-ened by negative statistics, they relied on prayer for strength and to help keep their fears under control.

> The first thing I did is to ask God to give me the strength so I could help my family when I tell them, and it wasn't as hard telling my husband, but it was very hard telling my daughters. And I couldn't tell my sons at all.

Alternatively, some participants experienced spiritual struggles in dealing with the physical and emotional challenges imposed by the illness. Overall, spiritu-ality and healthcare provider communication provided a context that influenced women's abilities to transform the death sentence.

Shock: Reverberating From the Impact

Sensing the threat: The shock phase consisted of three stages: sensing the threat, succumbing to the vortex, and surviving the chaos. During the initial stage leading up to the diagnosis, many women experienced vague symptoms and sensed that something was wrong but did not suspect cancer. Most women sought care from their primary providers, and a few sought specialist care. Although some women were satisfied with those interactions, many felt distressed because of misdiagnoses or delayed diagnoses that they believed contributed to being diagnosed at a more advanced stage. Unless significant physical findings existed, the diagnosis usually was missed initially either by the primary provider or the specialist. Although some were referred to a specialist immediately, several were treated symptomatically until symptoms worsened or they insisted on further workup.

> So all this pussyfooting around went on. I went back and forth with the doctor. Yes, I am in pain and no, I am not seeing anything or feeling anything or protecting anything. . . . Finally, by the time I got to the scheduled day of surgery of the gallbladder, I could hardly walk.

Women experienced other delays related to lack of coordination of follow-up appointments or when providers did not call to expedite referrals to specialists.

> I went for my annual Pap [examination] . . . and it came back abnormal. I ended up having to go several times because [of] scheduling problems with the office. . . . The doctor, again, wasn't there, and I finally said, "I've had it. I'll see anybody—whoever's there."

These concerns contributed to the distress experienced when the diagnosis was confirmed.

Succumbing to the vortex: Many women felt overwhelmed, scared, and traumatized on hearing the diagnosis.

> I thought I was going to die. I thought I was going to pass out. I was upset. I called my roommate and I was hysterical. I didn't know what to do. . . . I was like blown away. . . . It was a complete shock. . . . To me, ovarian cancer is a death sentence.

One woman was so upset that she was oblivious to the fact that she damaged her car in the parking lot.

> Well, I was so upset that morning, when I pulled up, I tore the whole right side off my car, because I was going to the doctor and I was just very upset. . . . I didn't realize what I had done till after I had done it.

Women experienced a whirlwind of activity as they prepared for upcoming surgery, and some women did not realize the impact until they had more time to process the news.

And I honestly think that, at the time, it actually hit my husband a lot harder than it hit me. I think that was because I was just so sick that I really just didn't think of it too much. . . . I was just feeling terrible and in so much pain that I didn't think too far in the future and I just wanted to feel better.

Surviving the chaos: Women managed the chaos by adopting various coping styles and control measures such as preparing for treatment and controlling the information about the disease. They controlled the information using somewhat contradictory strategies, including seeking and avoiding information. Women initially sought out information from various sources, including the Internet and their healthcare providers, but frequently felt threatened and reported mixed feelings related to the negative statistics.

I had sorta mixed emotions about that. If I came upon something that really said something about it, I wanted to read it. But I wasn't really looking for it. In the beginning, I was looking for information on it and like I said I was afraid if I started reading, after I started reading about different things, it sort of scared me.

Women relied on various coping styles such as fighting spirit, denial, minimization, and avoidance to help them manage the psychological impact. For example, some participants denied or minimized the significance of their illness.

You really don't [take the time to process that you had cancer]. You kind of deny it. . . . I'm fine, don't tell me I need to go home. . . . I think that's one way you can get through it.

Other participants avoided or selectively ignored information they perceived as threatening. The use of various control measures and coping styles helped women achieve a greater sense of control, which facilitated the transition to the next phase.

Aftershock: Grasping Reality

During the aftershock phase, participants were more introspective in recognizing their vulnerability and relied on various coping strategies as they struggled with the realization of a potentially limited future. The phase consisted of three stages: acknowledging the fear, mobilizing resources, and internalizing the illness.

Acknowledging the fear: several participants expressed that their biggest fear was recurrence and dying, described as "standing on shaky ground." Women reported feeling more anxious and scared at night, coined by one participant as the "danger zone."

Probably when I'm alone is the hardest. Alone with my thoughts because it allows me to think more and go to places that I don't really want to go to. . . . At night, when I lie down to go to sleep, it's probably the hardest time. Because my mind wanders; it goes places I don't want to go to.

Many participants expressed mixed feelings or anxiety after completing chemotherapy when no longer under the protection of cancer-fighting drugs.

[I felt] scared and fearful that every time he give me a pelvic or something that he will say, "Oh, something is not normal." . . . I even told my husband that I am scared. If I die, don't give all of my things away.

I guess the only thing that worries me is having less frequent checkups at the doctor's office, then trying to decide, based on symptoms, do I go in. . . . It is kind of comforting to go in on a predetermined schedule on dates that are not too far apart.

Conditions that influenced or delayed the process included functional limitations and significant life events such as stress related to a family crisis.

Mobilizing resources: Women mobilized resources and familiar coping strategies as they sought to regain control. They relied on inner strength, including prior challenging life events, which helped them to cope with the illness. Women also appraised their support systems in considering who would be most helpful for emotional or practical assistance and reached out to people who were optimistic and encouraging.

Sometimes I could talk very easily and comfortable with someone and share my innermost feelings. But I didn't want anyone weeping, upchucking, and really upset with what happened. . . . I wanted someone to say, "We will work at this together."

Many women were concerned about the impact of the illness on their families and considered their needs as they dealt with the illness. Some women tried to protect their families by minimizing their own fears or confiding in a close friend rather than a family member.

Although support was critical, it could be overwhelming at times, and women took steps to manage it. Women frequently relied on their husbands or a trusted friend to relay information or coordinate offers of help. Some participants actively avoided certain people who were negative or unsupportive in their communications.

There was a couple of people who called me and told me some negative things that made me sorta not feel so good. . . . I know I won't be talking to them for a while.

Many women received a significant source of support from other survivors. Although some actively sought out survivors, others feared that attending support groups or encountering others who were doing poorly would be a negative experience. However, those women were grateful for unexpected sources of support.

> It was like having these people in your life, coming to me and talking to me about it. It really helped, and I was really confident. It helped me realize that you can do it. Not just talking to somebody on the phone.

Internalizing the illness: Women looked back at the experience as being somewhat surreal and realized that their lives had changed completely. A few women referred to it as "stepping through the looking glass," an analogy from *Alice in Wonderland,* and described a feeling of being on the outside looking in, as if this were happening to someone else.

> You have to deal even [though] you know on some level, it's sort of like there's two people operating. You have to deal with it, but then sometimes it feels like somebody else is actually going through it. Yeah. I don't know whether that's just to escape it.

Women recognized the many losses and changes in their roles and relationships, including grief related to the realization of a potentially limited future.

> I think I have always looked to my kids that I was the rock. That I could do anything. . . . All of a sudden, it was like, it is not going to be always that way. . . . When I came home after seeing Dr. B that day, I pulled in my driveway . . . and cried uncontrollably. Because I said I finally found my house . . . and now I'm going to lose it.

The process of facing the poor prognosis occurred over time and involved struggling with uncertainty, fears, and loss of control. Women struggled to hold onto the belief that they would be okay while not being certain.

> I wanted to know right now if I was going to be okay. . . . The patience is hard. That made me shaky. You get through that. It was out of my control. It was difficult; I wanted it to be in my control.

Other participants described a turning point or pivotal event that helped them to face the poor prognosis, such as having a sudden realization upon encountering another young woman dying of cancer. Women's abilities to internalize the illness helped them to better manage the uncertainty and begin to rebuild their lives.

Rebuilding: Living the New Paradigm

Women continued to experience fears during the rebuilding phase but were coming to terms with the losses and learning to live with the uncertainty. The phase consisted of three stages: managing the uncertainty, shifting expectations, and searching for meaning. The transition generally occurred sometime after completing therapy, as participants had more time to reflect on their experiences.

Managing the uncertainty: Women relied on various coping styles to help them manage the underlying sense of uncertainty. They struggled with the reality that cancer may recur while trying to figure out how to go on with their lives, adopting an attitude of living one day at a time.

> You know 'cause you always want to be proactive and now you're in the wait-and-see mode. . . . But there's nothing you can do. . . . it's mostly trying to figure out how you go on with your life without dwelling on the fact that three months from now you are going to have an exam or . . . the blood work. . . . You can't—you just can't think that far in advance.

Women continued to rely on coping styles, including rationalization, minimization, humor, and social comparisons. Participants compared themselves to others in similar circumstances and engaged in downward and upward comparisons. For example, several participants compared themselves with long-term survivors, which provided inspiration and hope that they too could survive.

> So we were talking and she [a neighbor with ovarian cancer] just got her five-year mark. You talk about happy now, I was happy then I was really, really happy. . . . My feet weren't on the ground.

Maintaining positive alliances with survivors provided reassurance and great meaning to participants.

Shifting expectations: Several women revised their expectations and goals as they focused on meaningful priorities in their lives. The process occurred over time and involved accepting losses such as changing jobs or career goals or adjusting expectations related to the disease. Women focused on meaningful goals, such as returning to work and usual activities, because they wanted their lives to be normal again. However, the inability to return to one's normal activities was associated with decreased hope.

> Hope is just a realistic expectation of things getting better. That's what I gotta have. Not just a pie in the sky. . . . I want to get up and get around. . . . I want to resume a reasonably normal life. . . . I want to be able to control living and not just vegetate.

Searching for meaning: Women tried to move beyond their present circumstances to find meaning and a new perspective on life. Many focused on living day to day, expressed a renewed appreciation for life and close relationships, and were realistic yet optimistic about the future.

> I don't take anything for granted. I try to stop and enjoy, take things at a slower pace, and really enjoy and not just rush through everything. Enjoy watching the girls grow up, not just going through the motions every day but actually being there.

The process of searching for meaning occurred over time and involved reflection and examination of values and priorities. Some women found meaning through participation in clinical trials and several expressed a desire to help other survivors. Closer to treatment, many women sought to help others in some way but were uncertain how to fulfill that goal. However, women further out from treatment had more time to decipher how they could contribute. Developmental tasks and functional limitations affected the process, including constraints imposed by family and work obligations.

Dimensions and Associated Categories

In examining the phases of transforming the death sentence, perceived support and control emerged as dimensions of the core variable. Life-threatening illnesses are associated with loss of control, and efforts to regain control were evident during the phases (see **Table 2**). Support assisted women in focusing

Table 2   Strategies That Enhanced Control in Each Phase

Phase	Strategies
I	Seeking and controlling the information
	Preparing for treatment
	Coping styles such as fighting spirit, denial, and avoidance
II	Mobilizing resources and support
	Managing the support
	Relying on faith
	Preparing for the future
III	Rationalization; upward and downward comparisons
	Shifting expectations or goals
	Finding meaning through altruistic activities

on positive aspects and seemed to positively influence perceived control. However, unsupportive interactions with family or friends contributed to distress. For this group of women, perceived control seemed to play a greater role in the process of transforming the death sentence. Women who felt in control of their environments and confident in their ability to manage symptoms and other areas of their lives were more hopeful.

Four categories of the core variable were identified based on levels of support and perceived control (see **Table 3**). Women with greater levels of support and control were more hopeful and able to face the death threat, whereas those with lower levels were least hopeful (see **Table 4**). Although the categories were somewhat fluid, most women aligned with the "going it alone" and "waiting for the other shoe to drop" categories. Women who aligned with "trapped in the illness" generally perceived the least support and control related to the disease or their environments. Women aligned with "waiting for the other shoe to drop" had difficulty coping with the losses and changes, but some were able to regain control with the encouragement of close others. Women aligned with "going it alone" were somewhat stoic and frequently reached out for support through ovarian cancer list serves or other venues. Women aligned with "facing the death threat" focused on tasks such as positive reappraisal and finding meaning.

DISCUSSION

The study supports findings from other studies of women with ovarian cancer and reveals new insights regarding women's experiences in dealing with the disease. Women with ovarian cancer have reported fears related to uncertainty and the possibility of early death (Bowes et al., 2002; Ferrell et al., 2005; Howell, Fitch, & Deane, 2003; Thompson, 2005). Facing the death threat emerged as women's main concern, and the basic social process, or core variable, in dealing with the concern was transforming the death sentence. Progression through the phases was influenced by overarching contextual themes, including healthcare provider communication and spirituality. Support and control emerged as key dimensions of the core variable that influenced women's hope. Based on those dimensions, four categories were identified that characterized women's abilities to transform the death sentence.

Although not the main concern, hope was a strong underlying theme that influenced the ability to transform the death sentence. The relationship of hope to the substantive theory in the study is supported by other models in the literature such as the Hope Process Framework (Farran et al., 1995; Farran, Wilken, & Popovich, 1992), which addresses four key processes of hope

Table 3 Categories of Transforming the Death Sentence

Category	Characteristics	Support	Perceived Control	Example Quotations
Facing the death threat	Focusing on meaningful goals Living day to day Finding meaning in the experience	High	High	You're at least able to groan about getting up and going to a job that you love, so being able to live my daily life everyday consistently is incredibly hopeful for me. That fills up the jar as well. When I'm in touch with my new friends who are such an inspiration to me. Other survivors ahead of me. The fact that people look to me as their inspiration to survive, whether they've had the cancer or not. I don't believe that God's done with my life at this point. He has given me people to talk with. At the National Institutes of Health, this woman, she just let me go on about God and my life and she just kept asking me more questions. . . . I think that's what life is about is knowing God and his love for us—letting others know it.
Waiting for the other shoe to drop	Struggling with fears, uncertainty Relying on support to help reappraise the situation Control enhanced by supportive others	High	Low	For a couple of weeks there, I didn't do anything. I wasn't on the thing with the diet, the exercise, or anything. Nothing . . . I guess it is like when you have chemo, you're fighting to survive and then you have made it. Well, I was talking with my aunt last night and . . . it will be five years for her. She said, "I understand because it is like you wait for the other shoe to fall." It is interesting when you can meet somebody that understands what you are saying. I feel a bit like a failure even though a lot of people say you're a survivor. . . . Inside, I feel kind of different, and it's hard to share that. I just told my mom that the other night. She got really upset and told a friend of mine. She said, "I look at her as . . . being so strong, and I really can't get that she feels like a failure." It's taken a lot from me.

Going it alone	Low	High	Relying on inner strength, determination Reaching out for support	I was born at the height of the Depression. . . . You grew up quick. . . . You have to learn to go get what you want. And not to expect it. It builds character. I think it molds you one way or the other. I think it helped me through this [experience]. So that being the case, I didn't see the need, um, I probably had enough of the resources within me that I didn't have that need to have that talk with God yet. And could be that it wasn't my time to have it but the inner resources are just, I think that they just come from an unexplained place.
Trapped in the illness	Low	Low	Overwhelmed, uncertain about the future Significant symptoms, functional limitations Preoccupied with intrusive thoughts Difficulty seeing beyond present circumstances	The pain started to overwhelm me and control me. I couldn't ignore it, I couldn't function with it, and I couldn't move. It just wouldn't go away. . . . My feet kept me awake at night. If I kept my feet out from under [the blanket], it was not too good either. I am preoccupied with it. Well, I feel like this, being human, I mean, I know I pray, I pray daily, and then the next thing I know I'm thinking about the same. I said, Lord, just take this out of my thoughts, out of my mind, just make me be free from thinking. And I'll be fine for a while, and the next thing I know, it's back up in my head again. I say, "Lord I'm not going to deal with that."

Table 4   Relationship of Hope to the Dimensions and Categories of the Core Variable

Category	Level of Perceived Control	Level of Support	Level of Hope
Trapped in the illness	Low	Low	Low
Waiting for the other shoe to drop	Low	High	Wavering
Going it alone	High	Low	Moderate
Facing the death threat	High	High	High

(see **Table 5**). Although some overlap exists, the Hope Process Framework provides a general framework to compare the theory emerging from the study with existing research findings.

Experiential Process of Hope

Women experienced tremendous loss and devastation associated with ovarian cancer, and their hope fluctuated during the course of the illness (Farran et al., 1995; McGee, 1984). Women reported uncertainty, loss of control, and losses related to a limited future (Howell et al., 2003; Thompson, 2005) and social and work roles (Ferrell, Smith, Ervin, Itano, & Melancon, 2003; Howell et al.; Little, Jordens, Paul, Montgomery, & Philipson, 1998; Navarre, 2004). Women relied on various coping styles and strategies to enhance control and manage the uncertainty, including reaching out for support.

Relational Process of Hope

Support from family, friends, and other cancer survivors was a major theme in women's descriptions of hope. Women managed the support so that it did not become overwhelming and avoided negative people or situations that threatened their hope (see also Crooks, 2001). Other research supported that stress related to unsupportive interactions with family or friends contributes to psychological distress among patients with cancer (Ekman, Bergbom, Ekman, Berthold, & Mahsneh, 2004; Marlow, Cartmill, Cieplucha, & Lowrie, 2003; Norton et al., 2005). Social support plays an important role in reducing illness uncertainty and improving QOL (Sammarco, 2003). Women used coping styles such as social comparisons as one way to reduce their fears and uncertainty (see Breetvelt and Van Dam [1991] for discussion of Festinger's social comparison theory). Although studies suggest that downward comparison is most

Table 5   Processes of Hope

Process	Focus
Experiential (**H**ealth)	Relationship of hope to suffering and loss; determining the relationship between patients' health status and hope
Relational (**O**thers)	Importance of relationships in promoting hope during difficult experiences; assessment of patients' support system and available resources
Spiritual and transcendent (**P**urpose)	Purpose in life or religious and spiritual orientation; assessment of patients' source of hope, which may involve spiritual assessment and the meaning of spiritual or religious practices
Rational thought (**E**ngaging)	Assessment of goals; internal and external resources that support hope and actions to attain goals. Assessment of sense of control and ways to increase control to foster hope. Assessment of perception of time in relationship to hope

Note. Based on information from Farran et al., 1992, 1995.

prevalent among those with chronic illness (Bogart & Helgeson, 2000; Bowes et al., 2002), many women in the study were inspired when comparing themselves to other survivors who were living their lives. Other studies support that upward social comparisons inspire hope and motivation in patients with cancer (Salander, Bergenheim, & Henriksson, 1996; Thompson, 2005). Although some women avoided support groups, most were inspired by communicating with other ovarian cancer survivors. Other studies support that connecting with similar others (Navarre, 2004) and support group participation provide hope and optimism about the future (Ahlberg & Nordner, 2006; Sivesind & Baile, 1997). Furthermore, sharing feelings and fears with others who had "walked in their shoes" validates women's experiences and helps them to realize that they are not alone (Ferrell, Smith, Juarez, & Melancon, 2003).

Spiritual and Transcendent Process of Hope

Women reported that spiritual beliefs and affirming relationships were important to their sense of hope. Many women found meaning through spirituality and spiritual practices, which facilitate positive reappraisal during stressful situations (Folkman, 1997; Lin & Bauer-Wu, 2003). Other research supports that spirituality is a source of hope (Ferrell, Smith, Juarez, et al., 2003; Kennelly, 2001) and that hope is linked to purpose or meaning in life (Ballard et al., 1997; Bowes et al., 2002; Farran et al., 1992; Herth, 1991; Post-White et al., 1996). Searching for meaning is a common existential theme (Bowes et al.; Ferrell, Smith, Juarez, et al.; Sivesind & Baile, 1997) and involves reflection, reevaluation (Halstead & Hull, 2001; Skaggs & Barron, 2006), and development of new short-term goals (Bowes et al.). In the present study, the process occurred over time and involved assessment of personal resources and preferences within the context of women's social environments.

Rational Thought Process of Hope

Assessment of goals: Hope involves revising goals so they are flexible and realistic because people are more motivated to achieve attainable goals (Farran et al., 1992; Felder, 2004; Herth, 1990). Shifting expectations and setting realistic goals promote a sense of meaning and personal control (Folkman, 1997; Folkman & Greer, 2000; Folkman & Moskowitz, 2000; Rothbaum, Weisz, & Snyder, 1982; Thompson & Collins, 1995; Thompson & Kyle, 2000). Participants reflected on their priorities and focused on getting back to normal. However, most were uncomfortable planning long term, perhaps because of the uncertainty associated with a life-threatening illness. Other studies support that hope is associated with short-term goal-setting and living as normally as possible (Ahlberg & Nordner, 2006; Benzein, Norberg, & Saveman, 2001; Pilkington & Mitchell, 2004). For example, Ferrell, Smith, Ervin, et al. (2003) found that returning to work and normal roles provided a sense of achievement in overcoming cancer and regaining normalcy.

Assessment of control: Sense of control is important in maintaining hope (Bunston, Mings, Mackie, & Jones, 1995; Ersek, 1992; Farran et al., 1995; Flemming, 1997). Women described experiences that supported and threatened their sense of control. Controlling the information about ovarian cancer was a major strategy that helped women to manage their fears. Rees and Bath (2001) also reported that women sought information to facilitate decision making and regain control over an uncontrollable situation. Women in the current study also avoided certain threatening information. Brashers (2001) noted that avoiding information about long-term prognosis may be positive because it supports optimism. Furthermore, patients may be ambivalent about the amount of information they desire (Bowes et al., 2002; Hack, Degner, & Parker, 2005; Pilkington & Mitchell, 2004) and may prefer hearing information about diagnosis in stages (Bowes et al.; Fitch, Deane, Howell, & Gray, 2002) to cope with it in "manageable bytes" (Dickerson, Boehmke, Ogle, & Brown, 2006). Threats to control included negative communications and financial and social pressures such as job discrimination. Unanticipated symptoms and physical impairments also threatened sense of control (Lockwood-Rayermann, 2006; Norton et al., 2005). Other studies support that symptom distress interferes with the ability to attain meaningful goals (Lee, Cohen, Edgar, Laizner, & Gagnon, 2006) and is associated with decreased hope (Benzein et al., 2001; Bowes et al.; Bunston et al.; Chang & Li, 2002; Felder, 2004; Herth, 1990, 1992; Kennelly, 2001).

Study Limitations

In patients with chronic illness, more than one interview may be needed to cover the topic area (Charmaz, 1990, 2000). The constructivist approach emphasizes developing a relationship through sustained involvement with participants, consistent with the symbolic interactionist's emphasis on meaning that emerges through social interaction. Although only one interview was conducted, the investigator spent additional time establishing rapport during consent meetings. Prospectively addressing women's experiences and hope over time in relationship to different phases of the illness trajectory would be helpful for future studies (Herth & Cutcliffe, 2002b).

NURSING IMPLICATIONS

Healthcare Provider Communication

Communication style and relationship with healthcare providers were significant recurring themes that influenced hope. Research supports the importance of patients' relationships with providers in influencing QOL (Lockwood-Rayermann, 2006; Pilkington & Mitchell, 2004) and meeting communication and psychosocial needs (Hack et al., 2005; Henman, Butow, Brown, Boyle, & Tattersall, 2002; Kornblith et al., 1995; Salander, 2002). Although many women experienced supportive interactions, some reported significant distress related to isolated negative communications. Information delivery can be challenging because information-seeking behaviors are highly individualistic (Hack et al.; Rees & Bath, 2001), and these behaviors may be indirect, potentially causing confusion and communication of information that patients perceive as intrusive (Brashers, Goldsmith, & Hsieh, 2002). Healthcare providers can support women by being sensitive to their information goals (Brashers et al.; Hack et al.; Rees & Bath) within the context of an ongoing supportive relationship (Salander).

Several women reported distress related to diagnostic delays, especially during the diagnostic period. Other studies of ovarian cancer survivors reported similar concerns related to delayed diagnosis (Bowes et al., 2002; Ferrell, Smith, Cullinane, & Melancon, 2003; Ferrell, Smith, Juarez, et al., 2003; Fitch et al., 2002; Koldjeski, Kirkpatrick, Swanson, Everett, & Brown, 2005). Other newly diagnosed patients with cancer emphasized the importance of individualized communication within the context of a crisis process and being given timely follow-up appointments (Salander, 2002).

Education

Women reported limited knowledge regarding support services and most healthcare professionals did not offer information about community resources. Other studies have reported dissatisfaction with information regarding psycho-social and practical issues (Ferrell, Smith, Ervin, et al., 2003; Fitch, Gray, & Franssen, 2001). Because various studies have emphasized the need for peer support with women facing the same illness (Ahlberg & Nordner, 2006; Bowes et al., 2002; Ferrell, Smith, Ervin, et al.; Fitch et al., 2000; Thompson, 2005), development of an Internet-based tool kit would assist providers and women with locating support resources (see **Figure 3** for additional strategies).

Symptom Management

Women experienced significant distress and fears of recurrence at various time points. For example, women reported intermittent anxiety prior to periodic

---

Figure 3   Strategies to Facilitate Communication and Sense of Control

- Expedite timely follow-up appointments and referrals, especially during the diagnostic period.
- Provide options and encourage active involvement in decision making.
- Assess education needs and clarify information presented on Web sites or from other sources.
- Listen to concerns and balance the communication of information with the need to maintain hope.
- Provide information about community resources, support groups, ovarian cancer list serves and advocacy groups (e.g., Association of Cancer Online Resources; *Conversations*; Ovarian Cancer National Alliance, the National Ovarian Cancer Coalition).
- Refer women to and lead or colead support groups.
- Screen for psychosocial distress using brief screening measures and refer to appropriate services.

Note. Based on information from the Association of Cancer Online Resources, 2007; Conversations, 2006; Dickerson et al., 2006; Felder, 2004; Fitch, 2003; Henman et al., 2002; Lammers et al., 2000; National Comprehensive Cancer Network, 2007; Ovarian Cancer National Alliance, 2007; Pilkington & Mitchell, 2004; Salander, 2002; Wright et al., 2004.

checkups and increased vulnerability during milestones such as completion of therapy (Hoskins & Haber, 2000; Lee et al., 2006; Schaefer, Ladd, Lammers, & Echenberg, 1999). Other studies support that women experience fears of recurrence after completing therapy (Ekman et al., 2004), which leads to physical hypervigilance, including anxiety associated with experiencing vague symptoms (Thompson, 2005; Schaefer et al.). Brief screening measures completed in the clinic may help to identify women at increased risk for distress (Fitch, 2003; Kornblith et al., 1995; McCorkle et al., 2003). Research supports the benefits of intervention by advanced practice nurses in reducing distress in newly diagnosed women (McCorkle et al.).

Future Research

Further research is needed regarding ovarian cancer–specific interventions (Thompson, 2005) that include a group support component (Ahlberg & Nordner, 2006). Conceptual models, such as the Theoretical Model of Appraisal and Coping (Folkman & Greer, 2000), the Medical Crisis Counseling Model (Koocher & Pollin, 2001; Shapiro & Koocher, 1996), the Social Cognitive Transition Model (Brennan, 2001), and the Hope Process Framework (Farran et al., 1992, 1995), may provide a framework for nursing interventions because they focus on enhancing well-being, perceived support, and control. Furthermore, interventions that enhance sense of control may facilitate coping and hopefulness (Buckley & Herth, 2004; Bunston et al., 1995).

Because women experience considerable distress at various transition points, such as the time of diagnosis and recurrence (Ferrell et al., 2005; Fitch, Deane, & Howell, 2003; McCorkle et al., 2003), targeted interventions are needed to support women at critical points during the illness (Ferrell et al., 2005; Thompson, 2005). Research supports the benefits of a phased approach in delivering interventions that account for concerns over time (Hoskins, 2001; Hoskins & Haber, 2000; Krupnick, Rowland, Goldberg, & Daniel, 1993). Because women do not always perceive that they receive adequate support from family and friends (Ekman et al., 2004; Ferrell, Smith, Ervin, et al., 2003; Schaefer et al., 1999), including significant others in interventions may facilitate adjustment.

Successful interventions require flexibility (Targ & Levine, 2002) and consideration of patient preferences (Carlsson & Strang, 1996; Lee et al., 2006; Palmer, Kagee, Coyne, & DeMichele, 2004). Group support approaches include traditional in-person groups, complementary therapy groups, various Internet-based forums, and telephone and community-based interventions (Davis, Cohen, & Apolinsky, 2005). As a result of geographic, illness, and cost limitations, interest in alternative modalities for delivering support and education has increased (Wilmoth, Tulman, Coleman, Stewart, & Samarel, 2006).

Creative interventions, such as Internet- and telephone-based groups, may be more effective in reaching greater numbers of women because ovarian cancer is less common than breast and other cancers. The flexibility, convenience, and cost-effectiveness of the Internet, including Web-based support groups and nursing interventions, merit further research to assess the benefits (Dickerson et al., 2006; Winzelberg et al., 2003) and limitations of these forums (Im, Chee, Tsai, Lin, & Cheng, 2005; Winzelberg et al.). Searching for meaning and spirituality are common themes in the ovarian cancer population; therefore, including complementary therapies in intervention research may be desirable because they focus on well-being (Lengacher et al., 2006), spirituality, and finding innate meaning in situations (Targ & Levine; Taylor, 2005).

CONCLUSION

Women with ovarian cancer are vulnerable because of the unique challenges they face in the context of living with a life-threatening illness. Women with high levels of support and perceived control were best able to transform the death sentence and find meaning in the experience. Evidence-based interventions and strategies are needed to foster communication, symptom management, peer support, and spirituality. Holistic interventions that focus on enhancing support, perceived control, and hope should be a priority for future nursing research.

The author gratefully acknowledges the special women who generously shared their time and experiences and are applauded for being a source of hope, courage, and inspiration in helping other women facing ovarian cancer and advancing research in this area; her dissertation chair, Mary Elizabeth O'Brien, PhD, RN, FAAN; committee members, Janice Agazio, PhD, CRNP, RN, Marilyn Tuls Halstead, PhD, RN, AOCN®, and Elizabeth A. McFarlane, PhD, RN, FAAN; James F. Barter, MD, FACOG, and Jonathan A. Cosin, MD, FACOG, FACS, for their review and contribution to the study design; Patricia Goldman, president emeritus of the Ovarian Cancer National Alliance; and the nurses, doctors, and community leaders who helped facilitate this research. Special thanks are extended to Diane G. Cope, PhD, ARNP, BC, AOCNP®, for her thoughtful review and comments on this article.

REFERENCES

Ahlberg, K., & Nordner, A. (2006). The importance of participation in support groups for women with ovarian cancer [Online exclusive]. *Oncology Nursing Forum, 33,* E53–E61. Retrieved October 8, 2007, from http://ons.metapress.com/content/642190810204335/fulltext.pdf

Annells, M. (1996). Grounded theory method: Philosophical perspectives, paradigm of inquiry, and postmodernism. *Qualitative Health Research, 6,* 379–393.

Association of Cancer Online Resources. (2007). *OVARIAN homepage.* Retrieved April 16, 2007, from http://listserv.acor.org/archives/ovarian.html

Ballard, A., Green, T., McCaa, A., & Logsdon, M. C. (1997). A comparison of level of hope in patients with newly diagnosed and recurrent cancer. *Oncology Nursing Forum, 24,* 899–904.

Benzein, E., Norberg, A., & Saveman, B. I. (2001). The meaning of the lived experience of hope in patients with cancer in palliative home care. *Palliative Medicine, 15,* 117–126.

Blumer, H. (1969). *Symbolic interactionism: Perspective and method.* Englewood Cliffs, NJ: Prentice-Hall.

Bogart, L. M., & Helgeson, V. S. (2000). Social comparisons among women with breast cancer: A longitudinal investigation. *Journal of Applied Social Psychology, 30,* 547–575.

Bowes, D. E., Tamlyn, D., & Butler, L. J. (2002). Women living with ovarian cancer: Dealing with an early death. *Home Care for Women International, 23,* 135–148.

Brashers, D. E. (2001). Communication and uncertainty management. *Journal of Communication, 51,* 477–497.

Brashers, D .E., Goldsmith, D. J., & Hsieh, E. (2002). Information seeking and avoiding in health contexts. *Human Communication Research, 28,* 258–271.

Breetvelt, I. S., & Van Dam, F. S. (1991). Underreporting by cancer patients: The case of response-shift. *Social Science and Medicine, 32,* 981–987.

Brennan, J. (2001). Adjustment to cancer—Coping or personal transition? *Psycho-Oncology, 10,* 1–18.

Buckley, J., & Herth, K. (2004). Fostering hope in terminally ill patients. *Nursing Standard, 19*(10), 33–41.

Bunston, T., Mings, D., Mackie, A., & Jones, D. (1995). Facilitating hopefulness: The determinants of hope. *Journal of Psychosocial Oncology, 13*(4), 79–103.

Carlsson, M. E., & Strang, P. M. (1996). Educational group support for patients with gynaecological cancer and their families. *Supportive Care in Cancer, 4,* 102–109.

Cella, D. F. (1994). Quality of life: concepts and definition. *Journal of Pain and Symptom Management, 9,* 186–192.

Chang, L. C., & Li, I. C. (2002). The correlation between perceptions of control and hope status in home-based cancer patients. *Journal of Nursing Research, 10,* 73–81.

Charmaz, K. (1990). Discovering chronic illness: Using grounded theory. *Social Science and Medicine, 30,* 1161–1172.

Charmaz, K. (2000). Grounded theory: Objectivist and constructivist methods. In N.K. Denzin & Y. S. Lincoln (Eds.), *The handbook of qualitative research* (2nd ed., pp. 509–535). Thousand Oaks, CA: Sage.

Chi, G. C. (2007). The role of hope in patients with cancer. *Oncology Nursing Forum, 34,* 415–424.

Christopher, K. (2006). Older adults and cancer survivorship. In D.G. Cope & A.M. Reb (Eds.), *An evidence-based approach to the treatment and care of the older adult with cancer* (pp. 579–599). Pittsburgh, PA: Oncology nursing society.

Conversations. (2006). Retrieved April 16, 2007, from http://www.ovarian news.org/index.html

Crooks, D. L. (2001). Older women with breast cancer: New understandings through grounded theory research. *Health Care for Women International, 22,* 99–114.

Cutcliffe, J. (1996). Critically ill patients' perspectives of hope. *British Journal of Nursing, 5,* 674, 687–690.

Davis, C., Cohen, R., & Apolinsky, F. (2005). Providing social support to cancer patients: A look at alternative methods. *Journal of Psychosocial Oncology, 23,* 75–85.

Dickerson, S. S., Boehmke, M., Ogle, C., & Brown, J. K. (2006). Seeking and managing hope: Patients' experiences using the Internet for cancer care. *Oncology Nursing Forum, 33,* E8–E17.

Dufault, K., & Martocchio, B. (1985). Hope: Its spheres and dimensions. *Nursing Clinics of North America, 20,* 379–391.

Ekman, I., Bergbom, I., Ekman, T., Berthold, H., & Mahsneh, S. M. (2004). Maintaining normality and support are central issues when receiving chemotherapy for ovarian cancer. *Cancer Nursing, 27,* 177–182.

Ersek, M. (1992). The process of maintaining hope in adults undergoing bone marrow transplantation for leukemia. *Oncology Nursing Forum, 19,* 883–889.

Ersek, M., Ferrell, B. R., Dow, K. H., & Melancon, C.H. (1997). Quality of life in women with ovarian cancer. *Western Journal of Nursing Research, 19,* 334–350.

Farran, C. J., Herth, K. A., & Popovich, J. M. (1995). *Hope and hopelessness: Critical clinical constructs.* Thousand Oaks, CA: Sage.

Farran, C. J., Wilken, C., & Popovich, J. M. (1992). Clinical assessment of hope. *Issues in Mental Health Nursing, 13,* 129–138.

Felder, B. E. (2004). Hope and coping in patients with cancer diagnoses. *Cancer Nursing, 27,* 320–324.

Ferrell, B., Smith, S., Cullinane, C., & Melancon, C. (2003). Symptom concerns of women with ovarian cancer. *Journal of Pain and Symptom Management, 25,* 528–538.

Ferrell, B. R., Cullinane, C. A., Ervin, K., Melancon, C., Uman, G. C., & Juarez, G. (2005). Perspectives on the impact of ovarian cancer: Women's views of quality of life. *Oncology Nursing Forum, 32,* 1143–1149.

Ferrell, B. R., Smith, S. L., Ervin, K. S., Itano, J., & Melancon, C. (2003). A qualitative analysis of social concerns of women with ovarian cancer. *Psycho-Oncology, 12,* 647–663.

Ferrell, B. R., Smith, S. L., Juarez, G., & Melancon, C. (2003). Meaning of illness and spirituality in ovarian cancer survivors. *Oncology Nursing Forum, 30,* 249–257.

Ferrell, B. R., Virani, R., Smith, S., & Juarez, G. (2003). The role of oncology nursing to ensure quality care for cancer survivors: A report commissioned by the National Cancer Policy Board and Institute of Medicine [Online exclusive]. *Oncology Nursing Forum, 30,* E1–E11. Retrieved October 8, 2007, from http://ons.metapress.com/content/3k31602727q874h5/fulltext.pdf

Fitch, M., Deane, K., Howell, D., & Gray, R. E. (2002). Women's experiences with ovarian cancer: Reflections on being diagnosed. *Canadian Oncology Nursing Journal, 12,* 152–159.

Fitch, M. E., Deane, K., & Howell, D. (2003). Living with ovarian cancer: Women's perspectives on treatment and treatment decision-making. *Canadian Oncology Nursing Journal, 13,* 8–13.

Fitch, M. I. (2003). Psychosocial management of patients with recurrent ovarian cancer: Treating the whole patient to improve quality of life. *Seminars in Oncology Nursing, 19*(3, Suppl. 1), 40–53.

Fitch, M. I., Gray, R. E., & Franssen, E. (2000). Women's perspectives regarding the impact of ovarian cancer: Implications for nursing. *Cancer Nursing, 23,* 359–366.

Fitch, M. I., Gray, R. E., & Franssen, E. (2001). Perspectives on living with ovarian cancer: Older women's views. *Oncology Nursing Forum, 28,* 1433–1442.

Flemming, K. (1997). The meaning of hope to palliative care cancer patients. *International Journal of Palliative Nursing, 3,* 14–18.

Folkman, S. (1997). Positive psychological states and coping with severe stress. *Social Science and Medicine, 45,* 1207–1221.

Folkman, S., & Greer, S. (2000). Promoting psychological well-being in the face of serious illness: When theory, research and practice inform each other. *Psycho-Oncology, 9,* 11–19.

Folkman, S., & Moskowitz, J. T. (2000). Positive affect and the other side of coping. *American Psychologist, 55,* 647–654.

Glaser, B. G. (1978). *Theoretical sensitivity.* Mill Valley, CA: Sociology Press.

Glaser, B. G. (1992). *Basics of grounded theory analysis.* Mill Valley, CA: Sociology Press.

Glaser, B. G., & Strauss, A. L. (1967). *The discovery of grounded theory.* Chicago, IL: Aldine Publishing.

Guba, E. G., & Lincoln, Y. S. (1989). *Fourth generation evaluation.* Newbury Park, CA: Sage.

Hack, T. F., Degner, L. F., & Parker, P. A. (2005). The communication goals and needs of cancer patients: A review. *Psycho-Oncology, 14,* 831–845.

Halstead, M. T., & Hull, M. (2001). Struggling with paradoxes: The process of spiritual development in women with cancer. *Oncology Nursing Forum, 28,* 1534–1544.

Henman, M. J., Butow, P. N., Brown, R. F., Boyle, F., & Tattersall, M. H. (2002). Lay constructions of decision-making in cancer. *Psycho-Oncology, 11,* 295–306.

Herth, K. A. (1990). Fostering hope in terminally-ill people. *Journal of Advanced Nursing, 15,* 1250–1259.

Herth, K. A. (1991). Development and refinement of an instrument to measure hope. *Scholarly Inquiry for Nursing Practice, 5,* 39–51.

Herth, K. A. (1992). Abbreviated instrument to measure hope: Development and psychometric evaluation. *Journal of Advanced Nursing, 17,* 1251–1259.

Herth, K. A., & Cutcliffe, J. R. (2002a). The concept of hope in nursing III: Hope and palliative care nursing. *British Journal of Nursing, 11,* 977–983.

Herth, K. A., & Cutcliffe, J. R. (2002b). The concept of hope in nursing VI: Research/education/policy/practice. *British Journal of Nursing, 11,* 1404–1411.

Hoskins, C. N. (2001). Promoting adjustment among women with breast cancer and their partners: A program of research. *Journal of the New York State Nurses' Association, 32*(2), 19–23.

Hoskins, C. N., & Haber, J. (2000). Adjusting to breast cancer. *American Journal of Nursing, 100*(4), 26–32.

Howell, D., Fitch, M. I., & Deane, K. A. (2003). Impact of ovarian cancer perceived by women. *Cancer Nursing, 26,* 1–9.

Hutchinson, S. A., & Wilson, H. S. (2001). Grounded theory: The method. In P. Munhall (Ed.), *Nursing research: A qualitative perspective* (3rd ed., pp. 209–243). Sudbury, MA: Jones and Bartlett.

Im, E. O., Chee, W., Tsai, H. M., Lin, L. C., & Cheng, C. Y. (2005). Internet cancer support groups: A feminist analysis. *Cancer Nursing, 28,* 1–7.

Kennelly, L. F. (2001). Symptom distress, spirituality, and hope among persons with recurrent cancer. *Dissertation Abstracts International, 61*(10), 523B. (UMI No. 9992352).

Koldjeski, D., Kirkpatrick, M. K., Swanson, M., Everett, L., & Brown, S. (2005). An ovarian cancer diagnosis-seeking process: Unraveling the diagnostic delay problem. *Oncology Nursing Forum, 32,* 1036–1042.

Koocher, G. P., & Pollin, I. S. (2001). Preventive psychosocial intervention in cancer treatment. in A. Baum & B. L. Anderson (Eds.), *Psychosocial interventions for cancer* (pp. 363–374). Washington, DC: American Psychological Association.

Kornblith, A. B., Thaler, H. T., Wong, H., Vlamis, V., Lepore, J. M., Loseth, D. B., et al. (1995). Quality of life of women with ovarian cancer. *Gynecologic Oncology, 59,* 231–242.

Krupnick, J. L., Rowland, J. H., Goldberg, R. L., & Daniel, U. V. (1993). Professionally-led support groups for cancer patients: An intervention in search of a model. *International Journal of Psychiatry in Medicine, 23,* 275–294.

Lammers, S. E., Schaefer, K. M., Ladd, E. C., & Echenberg, R. (2000). Caring for women living with ovarian cancer: Recommendations for advanced practice nurses. *Journal of Obstetric, Gynecologic, and Neonatal Nursing, 29,* 567–573.

Lee, V., Cohen, S. R., Edgar, I., Laizner, A. M., & Gagnon, A. J. (2006). Meaning-making and psychological adjustment to cancer: Development of an intervention and pilot results. *Oncology Nursing Forum, 33,* 291–302.

Lengacher, C. A., Bennett, M. P., Kip, K. E., Gonzalez, L., Jacobsen, P., & Cox, C. E. (2006). Relief of symptoms, side effects, and psychological distress through the use of complementary and alternative medicine in women with breast cancer. *Oncology Nursing Forum, 33,* 97–104.

Lin, H. R., & Bauer-Wu, S. M. (2003). Psycho-spiritual well-being in patients with advanced cancer: An integrative review of the literature. *Journal of Advanced Nursing, 44,* 69–80.

Lincoln, Y. S., & Guba, E. G. (1985). *Naturalistic inquiry.* Beverly Hills, CA: Sage.

Lincoln, Y. S., & Guba, E. G. (2000). Paradigmatic controversies, contradictions, and emerging confluences. In N. K. Denzin & Y. S. Lincoln (Eds.), *Handbook of qualitative research* (2nd ed., pp. 163–188). Thousand Oaks, CA: Sage.

Little, M., Jordens, C. F., Paul, K., Montgomery, K., & Philipson, B. (1998). Liminality: A major category of the experience of cancer illness. *Social Science and Medicine, 47,* 1485–1494.

Lockwood-Rayermann, S. (2006). Survivorship issues in ovarian cancer: A review. *Oncology Nursing Forum, 33,* 553–562.

Marlow, B., Cartmill, T., Cieplucha, H., & Kowrie, S. (2003). An interactive process model of psychosocial support needs for women living with breast cancer. *Psycho-Oncology, 12,* 319–330.

McCorkle, R., Pasacreta, J., & Tang, S. T. (2003). The silent killer: Psychological issues in ovarian cancer. *Holistic Nursing Practice, 17,* 300–308.

McGee, R. F. (1984). Hope: A factor influencing crisis resolution. *Advances in Nursing Science, 6*(4), 34–44.

National Comprehensive Cancer Network. (2007). *NCCN clinical practice guidelines in oncology: Distress management* [v.1.2007]. Retrieved April 17, 2007, from http://www.nccn.org/professionals/physician_gls/PDF/distress.pdf

Navarre, S. E. (2004). Controlling vulnerability: Survival of middle-aged women with breast cancer. *Dissertation Abstracts International, 65*(4), 1782B. (UMI No. 3130855).

Norton, T. R., Manne, S. L., Rubin, S., Hernandez, E., Carlson, J., Bergman, C., et al. (2005). Ovarian cancer patients' psychological distress: The role of physical impairment, perceived unsupportive family and friend behaviors, perceived control, and self-esteem. *Health Psychology, 24,* 143–152.

Nowotny, M. L. (1989). Assessment of hope in patients with cancer: Development of an instrument. *Oncology Nursing Forum, 16,* 57–61.

Ovarian Cancer National Alliance. (2007). Retrieved April 16, 2007, from http://www.ovarian cancer.org

Palmer, S. C., Kagee, A., Coyne, J. C., & DeMichele, A. (2004). Experience of trauma, distress, and posttraumatic stress disorder among breast cancer patients. *Psychosomatic Medicine, 66,* 258–264.

Patton, M.Q. (1990). *Qualitative evaluation and research methods* (2nd ed.). Newbury Park, CA: Sage.

Payne, J. K. (2006). Research issues and priorities. In D. G. Cope & A. M. Reb (Eds.), *An evidence-based approach to the treatment and care of the older adult with cancer* (pp. 13–40). Pittsburgh, PA: Oncology Nursing Society.

Penrod, J., & Morse, J. M. (1997). Strategies for assessing and fostering hope: The hope assessment guide. *Oncology Nursing Forum, 24,* 1055–1063.

Pilkington, F. B., & Mitchell, G. J. (2004). Quality of life for women living with a gynecologic cancer. *Nursing Science Quarterly, 17*(2), 147–155.

Posluszny, D. M. (2001). Psychological trauma and adjustment in women newly-diagnosed with gynecologic cancer. *Dissertation Abstracts International, 62*(05), 2497B. (UMI No. 3013324).

Post-White, J., Ceronsky, C., Kreitzer, M., Nickelson, K., Drew, D., Mackey, K., et al. (1996). Hope, spirituality, sense of coherence, and quality of life in patients with cancer. *Oncology Nursing Forum, 23,* 1571–1579.

Rees, C. E., & Bath, P. A. (2001). Information-seeking behaviors of women with breast cancer. *Oncology Nursing Forum, 28,* 899–907.

Rothbaum, F., Weisz, J. R., & Snyder, S. S. (1982). Changing the world and changing the self. A two process model of perceived control. *Journal of Personality and Social Psychology, 42,* 5–37.

Rustoen, T. (1995). Hope and quality of life, two central issues for cancer patients: A theoretical analysis. *Cancer Nursing, 18,* 355–361.

Rustoen, T., & Hanestad, B. R. (1998). Nursing intervention to increase hope in cancer patients. *Journal of Clinical Nursing, 7,* 19–27.

Salander, P. (2002). Bad news from the patient's perspective: An analysis of the written narratives of newly diagnosed cancer patients. *Social Science and Medicine, 55,* 721–732.

Salander, P., Bergenheim, T., & Henriksson, R. (1996). The creation of protection and hope in patients with malignant brain tumors. *Social Science and Medicine, 42,* 985–996.

Sammarco, A. (2003). Quality of life among older survivors of breast cancer. *Cancer Nursing, 26,* 431–438.

Sandelowski, M. (1986). The problem of rigor in qualitative research. *Advances in Nursing Science, 8*(3), 27–37.

Schaefer, K. M., Ladd, E. C., Lammers, S. E., & Echenberg, E. J. (1999). In your skin you are different: Women living with ovarian cancer during childbearing years. *Qualitative Health Research, 9,* 227–242.

Shapiro, D. E., & Koocher, G. P. (1996). Goals and practical considerations in outpatient medical crises intervention. *Professional Psychology: Research and Practice, 27,* 109–120.

Sivesind, D., & Baile, W. (1997). An ovarian cancer support group. *Cancer Practice, 5,* 247–251.

Skaggs, B. G., & Barron, C. R. (2006). Searching for meaning in negative events: Concept analysis. *Journal of Advanced Nursing, 53,* 559–570.

Stern, P. N. (1980). Grounded theory methodology: Its uses and processes. *Image, 12*(1), 20–23.

Targ, E. F., & Levine, E. G. (2002). The efficacy of a mind-body-spirit group for women with breast cancer: A randomized controlled trial. *General Hospital Psychiatry, 24,* 238–248.

Taylor, E. J. (2005). Spiritual complementary therapies in cancer care. *Seminars in Oncology Nursing, 21,* 159–163.

Thompson, K. (2005). The phenomenology of loss: Interpersonal and intra-psychic experiences in women with ovarian cancer. *Dissertation Abstracts International, 65*(11), 4351A. (UMI No. 3154936).

Thompson, S. C., & Collins, M. A. (1995). Applications of perceived control to cancer: An overview of theory and measurement. *Journal of Psychosocial Oncology, 13*, 11–26.

Thompson, S. C., & Kyle, D. J. (2000). The role of perceived control in coping with the losses associated with chronic illness. In J. Harvey & E. D. Miller (Eds.), *Loss and trauma: General and close relationship perspectives* (pp. 131–145). Philadelphia, PA: Brunner-Routledge.

Wilmoth, M. C., Tulman, L., Coleman, E. A., Stewart, C. B., & Samarel, N. (2006). Women's perceptions of the effectiveness of telephone support and education on their adjustment to breast cancer. *Oncology Nursing Forum, 33*, 138–144.

Winzelberg, A. J., Classen, C., Alpers, G. W., Roberts, H., Koopman, C., Adams, R. E., et al. (2003). Evaluation of an Internet support group for women with primary breast cancer. *Cancer, 97*, 1164–1173.

Wolcott, H. F. (2002). Writing up qualitative research . . . better. *Qualitative Health Research, 12*, 91–103.

Wright, E. B., Holcombe, C., & Salmon, P. (2004). Doctors' communication of trust, care, and respect in breast cancer: Qualitative study. *BMJ, 328*, 864. Retrieved March 3, 2006, from http://bmj.bmjjournals.com/cgi/reprint/328/7444/864

Anne M. Reb, PhD, NP, is a research nurse manager at the Henry M. Jackson Foundation, United States Military Cancer Institute, in Washington, DC. Funding for this study was provided by the ONS Foundation and an Oncology Nursing Certification Corporation research grant. (Submitted April 2007. Accepted for publication June 8, 2007.)

Author Contact: Anne M. Reb, PhD, NP, may be contacted at areb@comcast.net, with copy to the editor at OnFEditor@ons.org.

A Place to be Yourself: Empowerment from the Client's Perspective

LYNNE M. CONNELLY, BECKY S. KEELE,
SUSAN V. M. KLEINBECK,
JOANNE KRAENZLE SCHNEIDER,
ANN KUCKELMAN COBB

This article describes a focused ethnography of a group of chronically mentally ill clients who were involved in a client-run drop-in center. Spradley's (1979) Developmental Research Sequence guided the research. Data were obtained from interviews, participant-observation and documents review. The qualitative analysis identified the major theme of empowerment, which had four process domains: participating, choosing, supporting and negotiating. These domains represented four levels of empowerment for this group. From the clients' perspective, empowerment meant they participated more in the community, their choices were increased, they provided support for each other and they negotiated on a more equal basis with staff. A fifth domain, personal significance, described the effects of empowerment for each individual.

Since consumer involvement in decision-making has been mandated recently by law (Mental Health Act Amendments of 1990), health care providers have had to reexamine the way services are delivered. Clients are being asked for their input and many are taking the initiative in developing client-run programs.

SOCIAL CONTEXT OF THE STUDY

The project was conducted in a suburban county mental health center in the Midwest. The center's community support services (CSS) unit serves over 400 county residents who have serious and persistent mental illness, primarily schizophrenia and maniac-depression. The mission of CSS is to assist

From "A place to be yourself: Empowerment from the client's perspective," by L. M. Connelly, B. S. Keele, S. V. Kleinbeck, J. K. Schneider, & A. K. Cobb, 1993, *Journal of Nursing Scholarship*, 25(4), 297–303. Copyright 2003 by John Wiley and Sons. Reprinted with permission.

individuals toward success in living, learning and working in the social environ-ments of their choice. It provides a variety of residential and supported hous-ing options, vocational services, group therapy, skills building and social and educational programs. Emergency services are available 24 hours a day.

In response to the Mental Health Act Amendments of 1990 and the corre-sponding state laws for implementation, CSS staff developed a philosophy that actively supports client involvement in decision-making. In the fall of 1990, a group of CSS clients asked to organize a client-run drop-in center. Previously there had only been a small waiting room where clients could sit, smoke and talk. This waiting room was an open area where it was difficult to carry on a personal conversation. The clients wanted a place of their own, where staff would be al-lowed only by invitation. With the support of CSS staff, the clients met to develop the goals and purposes of the drop-in center. A client board of seven directors was formed to oversee the design and on-going operations of the center. The clients held a contest and named the center Prairie Place (a pseudonym).

The staff noted that clients who had shown little initiative in the past began taking on responsibility, acting more assertively and requesting additional re-sources to accomplish further goals. They asked to become van drivers and to hold client-only parties after hours in the drop-in center. These changes produced some trepidation on the part of staff, requiring some negotiation to work out the concerns of both groups.

CSS staff saw the changes in the clients as positive, but they had little time to study the effects in detail. Thus, they welcomed the possibility of a group research project to be conducted by four doctoral students under the direction of a faculty advisor. A group approach was chosen because it increased the amount of data that could be gathered in one semester.

THE COMMUNITY MENTAL HEALTH MOVEMENT

The last four decades have been a time of hope and disappointment for the mentally ill. The community mental health movement began in the late 1940s (Morrissey & Goldman, 1986), with new developments in mental health care including psychotropic drugs and new therapeutic treatment techniques. By 1965, Congress passed Public Law 88-164, the Community Mental Health Centers (CMHC) Act, with amendments in 1965. These acts allocated funds for the construction and operation of comprehensive community-based mental health centers. However, the efforts to provide effective community care did not keep pace with the discharge of patients from mental hospitals throughout the 1960s and '70s. Originally CMHC programs were directed at the preven-tion of mental illness and care of less ill patients. As an increasing number of patients moved from long-term facilities into communities, CMHCs were faced with a growing population of chronically, seriously ill, socially impaired clients, for whom the system was not prepared (Morrissey & Goldman, 1986). For some 20 years, CMHCs struggled to provide services despite the lack of adequate funding.

Recently enacted legislation is a significant change in federal strategy. Public Law 99-660, the Comprehensive Mental Health Service Act (CMHS) of 1986 and the Mental Health Act Amendments of 1990, require states to plan and implement a comprehensive, community-based program of care for seriously mentally ill individuals as a condition for receiving Alcohol, Drug Abuse and Mental Health (ADM) block grants. The CMHS Act mandated participation and advice of consumers, their families, the mental health community and appropriate state agencies. Client rights groups have felt encouraged by the law because it is one of the first pieces of national legislation to mandate consumer involvement (Chamberlain & Rogers, 1990).

An excellent full-scale ethnography of a group of chronically mentally ill clients at a CMHC is Estroff's (1981) study, which provided background for the current project. It included a year and one-half of nearly continuous participant-observation, describing with great depth and sensitivity the difficulties encountered by the chronically mentally ill as they try to negotiate the everyday conflicts between the "normals" and the "crazies" who make up their world.

Clients in the setting described by Estroff were not affected by the recent changes mandating consumer participation as were the respondents in our study. It was this particular change on which we focused. Following the principle of emergent design (Lincoln & Guba, 1985) in qualitative research while restricting our focus to the effects of consumer participation in the CSS setting, we asked the following initial questions: 1) What is the clients' perspective of the factors that make the drop-in center successful? and 2) Do clients perceive themselves as having more power to make decisions than they had before the drop-in center was started? It was during the course of the study that empowerment emerged as a client theme.

METHODOLOGY

Design

Focused ethnography was chosen to describe the experience of the effects, from the client's perspective, of increased consumer participation in decision-making at the mental health drop-in center. Ethnography describes a culture or cultural scene in the "native" language (Spradley, 1979). The goal of ethnography is to grasp the subject's point of view; to see things from his or her unique place in the world. It offers an opportunity to systematically observe client life ways and patterns (Leininger, 1985) in a holistic manner (Germain, 1986).

Setting

The cultural scene (Spradley & McCurdy, 1982) studied in this project was the client run drop-in center, Prairie Place, that opened in December 1990. Prairie Place is located in the redesigned bottom floor of an office complex. Upon entering, there is an open area with chairs lining the perimeter, a kitchen nook, a resource and education room and an office for clients who are paid a minimal salary to serve as activity coordinators. Generally, several clients are sitting or standing, smoking and drinking coffee or iced tea. The atmosphere ranges from one that is quiet and relaxed to one of high activity and interaction.

Four client coordinators are employed part time at Prairie Place. Each works about 11 hours a week for $5 an hour and is responsible for keeping daily attendance records, planning the activities budget and scheduling activities. The latter include both indoor and outdoor events, such as Friday night parties, interagency volley ball leagues, picnics and local entertainment. The coordinators report to a board of seven client-elected directors. The board meets once a week and is responsible for the overall approval of plans, activities and finances.

DATA COLLECTION

Following approval from the human subjects committee, the research group made an initial entry into the setting by attending a Prairie Place client board meeting, where the purpose of the research was explained and participant-observation and interviewing was begun. The board members and staff in attendance were told that we were students in a doctoral program in nursing, and that we had two goals: to gain skill in conducting qualitative research, and to learn how the clients organize and manage services for themselves at a drop-in center like Prairie Place.

Data were collected over a five-week period. We chose informants with particular knowledge about the history and evolution of Prairie Place in order to obtain as detailed a picture as possible in a limited amount of time. We also chose a few clients who used the center but were not actively involved with running it to give a more complete perspective.

Twelve client informants and four professional staff who worked closely with the people involved were interviewed. The clients included board members, client coordinators and consumers who frequented Prairie Place. The interviews took approximately an hour, detailed field notes were handwritten during the interactions and transcribed as soon as possible after contact. Audio and videotaping were excluded as data collection methods to reduce intrusiveness with this relatively vulnerable population. Examples of questions that guided the interviews were: "What is it about Prairie Place that brings you here?" and "How are decisions made by consumers at Prairie Place?" The questions were broad initially to encourage the informants to share their experiences in their own words. The investigators followed the lead of the informants in exploring areas that were relevant to the questions.

Additional data collection methods included participant observation and document review. The focus of the participant-observation was to accurately describe the cultural scene and document decision-making as it occurred in the setting. Each of us attended at least one client board of directors meeting and several of the weekly client community meetings. As much time as our class schedules allowed was spent at Prairie Place. For example, time before and after interviews was spent there, talking with whomever was present. On one occasion, two of the researchers helped to decorate the center for a Halloween party. Another investigator was present during a tour of Prairie Place by a family member advocacy group. Notes of the participant-observations including informal conversations were written up as soon as possible after the observation. Documents reviewed were CSS brochures, newspaper articles, letters that the clients had written to the board, client-made posters and buttons.

To avoid observer bias and to ensure trustworthiness, data and investigator triangulation was used (Duffy, 1987). Debriefing among individual investigators as well as with the faculty advisor was also used (Lincoln & Guba, 1985). Member-checking was conducted by returning to selected informants and reviewing the domains we had identified, to see if the clients agreed or disagreed with our analysis. The final results were also reviewed with the clients in the form of a short oral presentation and a two page written report to the board.

Data Analysis

We conducted preliminary analysis of the data as it was being collected in order to generate working hypotheses that could be further explored. Data were analyzed using Spradley's (1979) Developmental Research Sequence. We initially each coded separately our own field notes using clients' original terms, key phrases and statements. Data were then pooled to total 36 informant domains which were comprised of six different semantic relationships. After considerable group discussion and debate, the initial domains were reformulated into five major domains with empowerment identified as the dominant theme. Four domains emerged that represented the components of the process of empowerment. The cover terms were participating, choosing, supporting and negotiating. The fifth domain was given the cover term "personal significance" and represented the effects of empowerment and its meaning for individual clients.

A systematic search for attributes was achieved through a componential analysis (**Table 1**). As attributes were identified, an ordering appeared among the domains. We saw the four process domains as levels of empowerment and the personal significance domain as the effects of empowerment on the individual. The raw data were reanalyzed to test the fit of the empowerment process and the ordering of domains. At this point, the literature on empowerment was reviewed for relevance to our study.

Table 1   Attributes of Empowerment

Participating	Choosing	Supporting	Negotiating	Personal Significance
Involvement	Options	Caring	Approximating equality	Meaning of empowerment to individual
	Freedom	Relating	Respecting	
	Self-control	Coaching	Cooperating	
	Courage	Accepting	Taking a Position	
		Sharing		

THE CONCEPT OF EMPOWERMENT

The term empowerment has been applied to a wide range of phenomena. It has been the focus of women's, Black power and gay rights movements (Minkler & Cox, 1980); the disabled elderly (Cohen, 1990); the chronically mentally ill (Zinman, 1982; Tobias, 1990; Bowler, 1991; Moxley, 1990); nurses (Mason et. al, 1990); the hospice patient/family (Bailey, 1990); local and global community change (McMurray, 1991); the student (Bough, 1991); the patient's rights movement (Zinman, 1982) and human services in general (Hasenfeld & Cheder, 1989).

Definitions of Empowerment

In psychology, Rappaport (1984), introduced the concept of empowerment to stimulate and guide mental health social policies. He defined empowerment broadly as a process by which people, organizations and communities gain mastery over their own lives. In nursing, Gibson (1991) redefined empowerment as a social process of recognizing, promoting and enhancing clients' abilities to meet their own needs, solve their own problems, and mobilize the necessary resources in order to feel in control of their own lives.

Empowerment as an Intervention Strategy

These definitions have served as the basis for empowerment as an intervention strategy in mental health settings. For example, Chesler (Hasenfeld & Chesler, 1989) encouraged peer counseling, organized support systems, and self-help groups as ways to empower families. Zinman (1982) called for client involvement in decision-making at all levels of the mental health institution, but argued that the first step towards empowerment is to raise the consciousness of a group to believe they are capable of running their own services and lives. Moxley and Freddolino's (1990) model of advocacy is similar to empowerment in that clients are encouraged to make their own decisions and to experience the consequences of these decisions as a means of moving toward independence.

Barriers to Empowerment

Barriers to empowerment are found at the societal, professional and client levels. For example, professionals' own lack of empowerment in the work setting and their inability and that of organizations to relinquish power affect client empowerment. Clients' lack of knowledge of strategies to promote empowerment, the negative effects of institutionalization, such as staff labeling, client dependency, apathy and distrust, are also disempowering. A third kind of barrier is social labeling which devalues client's feelings, ideas, values and beliefs (Hasenfeld & Chesler, 1989).

Research on Empowerment

Research related to empowerment has been varied, complex and multidisciplinary in nature, focusing on both micro and macro levels of society. Areas that have been studied include empowerment of citizens (Keiffer, 1984), the elderly in a community setting (Gallant, Cohen, & Wolff, 1985), nursing home residents (Langer & Rodin, 1970), a religious community (Maton & Rappaport, 1984) and a small American Indian community (O'Sullivan, Waugh, & Espeland, 1984). The failure of empowerment efforts has been studied in an alternative high school (Gruber & Trickett, 1987).

Nurse investigators have studied the empowerment of nurses related to autonomy in practice (Chandler, 1991; Collins & Henderson, 1991), and midwifery care (Morten, Kohl, O'Mahoney, & Pelosi, 1991) was studied as a means to empower clients and families. Nurse researchers have identified the dialogue between researcher and informant as empowering influence for women with diabetes (Anderson, 1991) and abused pregnant women (Parker & McFarlane, 1991). In a qualitative study of clients involved in a cardiac rehabilitation program (Flewy, 1991), "empowering potential" was found to be the process individuals used to maintain positive health behaviors.

A few studies have addressed empowerment of people with mental illnesses. In a study of community adaptation of recently discharged psychiatric patients (Joyce, Staley, & Hughes, 1990), comments made by informants suggested that a sense of control was important to preventing re-hospitalization. Interventions based on an empowerment model (Biegel, 1984) were implemented and studied in two urban ethnic neighborhoods over a four year period.

Self-help and support systems were developed in conjunction with community mental health centers and other human services. Rappaport et al. (1985) have conducted a study of a large mutual help organization for former psychiatric patients. The longitudinal nature of this collaborative study allowed the investigators to document the transformation of a subset of the organization's members from help seekers to help givers. We found no studies that investigated the process and meaning of empowerment from the perspective of individuals with chronic mental illness. Wallerstein (1992) and Rappaport (1984) have advocated the use of qualitative research methods including ethnography to study empowerment.

RESULTS AND DISCUSSION

In the process of analyzing the data for this study, a definition of empowerment was developed that is a modification of a definition by Gibson (1991). Empowerment is defined as a process wherein people assert control over the factors which affect their lives. The assumption is made that professional groups cannot empower clients, only the clients can empower themselves; however, health care providers can support clients and remove as many obstacles to empowerment as possible. This definition is similar to others (Bailey, 1990; Ingram, 1988; Malin & Teasdale, 1991; Tobias, 1990). The process of empowerment is on-going and involves levels through which individuals progress. The personal significance of empowerment varies with the individual and the level of empowerment at which the person is functioning.

The four levels of empowerment—participating, choosing, supporting and negotiating—describe the process that we observed with these clients. Clients at the first level of empowerment reported participating more than they previously had. At the second level, clients were choosing and experiencing the consequences of their choices. At the next level, clients were supporting and helping each other, moving beyond their internal world. At the negotiating level, clients reported interacting on a more equal basis with staff and each other in order to meet their needs. Each level subsumes the previous levels; therefore if someone is at the supporting level they also will be participating and choosing.

Participating

Participating, the initial level of empowerment, can simply be coming to the drop-in center. The only attribute of participating is involvement in Prairie Place. One of the clients said that for some people it's a big step to come to the center. In describing Prairie Place many clients said "It's a place to go." In a news article about Prairie Place, a client was quoted as saying that what Prairie Place "provides for clients is a convenient (place) where they are free to smoke, drink coffee, socialize and listen to music . . ." (Maag, 1991).

Support for this level was found in the literature. Participation is the beginning of reconnection to others and the creation of meaning in the lives of those involved (Haney, 1988). Rappaport (1984) commented that participation of people in their own empowerment is essential. Kieffer (1984) considered empowerment a long-term process that involves the development of participatory skills.

Choosing

Movement from the participating to the choosing level of empowerment varies with each person. Individuals at the choosing level are also participating. One client supported the simultaneous occurrence of these two levels:

> "I don't feel imprisoned. I have a lot of choices. You find out what the individual agrees to take part in. Participation, that's empowerment" (field notes).

Choosing implies that people have *freedom* to choose among various *options*. Having the courage to choose, they take control of their lives:

> "We want to solve problems ourselves, take control of our lives. Choices include classes in cooking, transportation, drawing, and exercise; whether to live in an apartment, Section VIII housing, or live in a group home" (field notes).

One attribute of choosing is *self-control*. Inherent in self-control is the assumption of responsibility for one's actions. This was reflected in a comment by one informant:

> "I mean staff will walk up and ask if I'll do something, and I have the right to say yes or no. If I say yes then I have the responsibility to do it" (field notes).

The literature supports choosing as an integral part of empowerment. Empowerment can be viewed as a synthesis of personal choice and social responsibility (Gibson, 1991). LaBonte (1989) pointed out that the origin of the word power is the Latin "potere"—the ability to choose. "We cannot empower anybody, because to presume to do so strips people of their ability to choose." People can only empower and motivate themselves. Bailey (1990) stated that one way to enhance feelings of empowerment is to accept and acknowledge responsibility for one's feelings, actions and choices.

Supporting

Supporting is the third level of the empowerment process. Attributes of this level include caring, relating, accepting, coaching and sharing. The following is an example of a client at the supporting level, demonstrating the attributes of *caring, relating, coaching* and *sharing* with another client:

> "I coached him on how to handle the situation. I showed him how to clean the range up, wipe it down and clean the pans . . . I show them an easier way. It's my job and I take care of them, so they can be better" (field notes).

Many other clients described how clients helped each other by listening, giving suggestions, visiting when someone was sick and just being friends. Friendship was very important to the people at Prairie Place.

An example of *accepting* as an attribute of the supporting level was given by an acutely ill client who, when asked how clients helped each other, said, "They talk to you. They accept your illness, even if you are real sick." Another informant stated that clients feel safe among their peer group.

Kieffer (1984) provided support for this domain, saying that empowerment is a transactional concept because the process involves a relationship with others. Where people are interrelated there is a sharing of resources, and collaboration is encouraged. Empowerment involves a person's ability to deal successfully with others and in the case of mentally ill clients, it frequently involves helping others. As individuals feel more empowered, they can draw on their inner resources to aid others to draw on theirs (Bailey, 1990).

Negotiating

The fourth level of empowerment is negotiating. Mutual *respect,* feelings of *near equality* and *cooperation* are identified as attributes of this level. In addition, clients frequently will *take a stand* on issues they consider important. One client leader stated:

> "I was the only one working at all. So I challenged them to start doing something . . . That all they were doing was coming to the center and smoking. 'Why don't you want to be a whole person?' I asked them. The community makes you feel like a whole person again. If I stay home and I don't volunteer or I don't help anybody to do anything then, to me, I'm not a whole person when I'm only thinking of myself" (field notes).

Clients negotiated to start Prairie Place; they helped design the building layout and the remodeling. They negotiated with the staff to maintain their own budget. The staff reached an agreement with the client committee allowing the clients to use space for Prairie Place. Another client described an incident that reflects the more complex level of negotiating:

> "I said 'why can't we go to the ball game?' and he [staff person] said, 'I'll leave this to you to do. You write the letter and ask the [pro-team] for the tickets.' I thought about it for a little while and decided I would give it a try . . . and two other clients helped me write the letter" (field notes).

External validation for this domain is provided by Hess (1984), who describes empowerment as a dynamic concept in which power is both taken and given. In other words, when the powerless exert pressure, the powerful may have to relinquish some control. This implies the idea of negotiation, where people are on a more equal footing and have certain rights.

Personal Significance

This domain reflects the participants' perceptions of the effects of moving through the process of empowerment. Our working hypothesis is that it differs from person to person and probably will differ with the same individual over time. Additional time in the field is required to identify these patterns as they change over time.

When we asked our informants to describe what benefits or results had occurred since Prairie Place opened, these various comments were made: I feel important; it keeps you out of the hospital; self-esteem; helping people regain control; understanding each other. One client felt that her involvement with patients' rights activities and Prairie Place had helped her become "almost well." Other words that clients used to describe empowerment were freedom, liberty, courage and responsibilities. Some described feelings of increased self-worth and confidence. Others reported feeling good or better about themselves. One client called empowerment "being an adult."

Empowerment can, however, have a negative effect on clients. Some clients felt stressed and overloaded because of increased responsibilities. Some clients had to quit volunteer positions on the board of directors because of perceived stress. One of the professional staff members said that before, clients became stressed because decisions were being made for them, and now they are stressed because they are making their own decisions. As empowerment is encouraged for mentally ill clients, health care providers must be aware of this possibility. As nurses, we can assist clients in working through any negative effects of the empowerment process, and we must guard against using this as an excuse to try to disempower them.

MODEL OF EMPOWERMENT

Although a focused ethnography does not usually involve development of a model, we found one useful in our understanding of empowerment for this group of clients. The two initial levels of empowerment (participating, choosing) represent an intrapersonal perspective or individual functioning. Individuals are operating to better their own situation and are primarily focused on themselves. The two higher levels of empowerment (supporting, negotiating) represent an interpersonal perspective, where a person is becoming more other-oriented. Empowered individuals at these levels are dealing more actively with and for other people. The personal significance domain conceptualizes the effects of the four process domains from the perspectives of participants in the empowerment process.

On completing our analysis and model, the literature was reviewed for support of the model. Kieffer's (1984) four stages of empowerment were similar to our levels, but there are some important differences. In his first stage, "era of entry," individuals participate at an exploratory level, where they are unsure and learning. This can be related to our level of "participating," which we see as a basic level of beginning involvement.

The next stage outlined by Kieffer is the "era of advancement," which is characterized by mentoring relationships and supportive peer relationships. This stage appears to relate more to our third level of empowerment, supporting. We believe there is a level that is characterized by choosing, i.e., being able to make successful choices for oneself. Perhaps this level reflects the challenges that Prairie Place clients face every day due to their illnesses. Having choices and dealing with the results is a very important part of empowerment.

Our third level, supporting, relates well to Kieffer's second "era of advancement" stage. The data demonstrate many ways that clients help each other to deal with life and mental illness. The third era, as outlined by Kieffer, is incorporation, which focuses on confronting and coming to grips with barriers to self-determination. This provides support for our fourth level of negotiation. Leadership skills are developed and clients learn to be assertive and more responsible for themselves and for Prairie Place.

Kieffer's fourth stage is the "era of commitment," where individuals integrate the skills they have learned into everyday life. In our analysis, we took a different view of commitment. Commitment occurred at all levels for the clients we observed. For some clients, just coming regularly to the center was a commitment at their level of functioning. For others who were more empowered, to come every day would be negative, because they would not be participating in the larger community. Commitment was different for each client, and even different for the same client at different times.

In our model, empowerment is viewed as levels rather than stages. As an individual moves along the levels, there is an increase in empowerment. There are no discrete stages, but an overlapping of the various levels. It is also possible to move along the continuum in both directions. The group of people we studied are challenged by periodic and severe episodes of mental disorganization and disorientation. During these acute phases, the client may operate at earlier levels of empowerment, and may require more active assistance with daily living. After the episode, a person may regain the previous level of empowerment. As Moxley and Freddolino (1990) pointed out, mental health clients face very real environmental challenges, barriers and resource problems in attaining their preferences largely because of discrimination, stigmatization, and lack of support. The level of empowerment of chronically mentally ill people cannot be compared to some norm, but must be viewed from the person's unique perspective at a particular time in life and with regard to his or her mental health.

In comparing our model with others, some similarities were found, but some significant differences were also evident. Many authors have addressed the idea of empowerment, but few have actually tried to present the clients' perspective. If empowerment of people is a desirable goal, then further study of the clients' perspective is in order. We cannot hope to be advocates for clients unless we know what they want and how they view empowerment.

REFERENCES

Anderson, J. M. (1991). Reflexivity in fieldwork: Toward a feminist epistemology. *Image: Journal of Nursing Scholarship, 23,* 115–118.

Bailey, B. L. (1990). The concepts of empowerment and care of the hospice patient and family. *Journal of Home Health Care Practitioner, 3*(1), 16–22.

Biegel, D. E. (1984). Help seeking and receiving in urban ethnic neighborhoods: Strategies for empowerment. *Prevention in Human Services, 3*(2/3), 37–71.

Bloche, M. G., & Cournos, F. (1990). Mental health policy for the 1990s: Tinkering in the interstices. *Journal of Health Politics, Policy and Law, 12,* 387–411.

Bough, S. (1991). A women's health course with a feminist perspective: Learning to care for and empower ourselves. *Nursing and Health Care, 12,* 76–80.

Bowler, J. B. (1991). Transformation into a healing health care environment: Recovering the possibilities of psychiatric/mental health nursing. *Perspectives in Psychiatric Care, 27*(2), 21–25.

Chamberlain, J., & Rogers, J. A. (1990). Planning a community-based mental health system. *American Psychologist, 45,* 1241–1244.

Chandler, G. E. (1991). Creating an environment to empower nurses. *Nursing Management, 22*(8), 20–23.

Cohen, E. (1990). The elderly mystique: Impediment to advocacy and empowerment. *Generations: Autonomy and Long-term Care,* Supplement, 13–16.

Collins, S. S., & Henderson, M. C. (1991). Autonomy: A part of the nursing role. *Nursing Forum, 26*(2), 23–29.

Duffy, M. E. (1987). Methodological triangulation: A vehicle for merging quantitative and qualitative research methods. *Image: Journal of Nursing Scholarship, 19,* 130–133.

Estroff, S. E. (1981). *Making it crazy: An ethnography of psychiatric clients in an American community.* Berkeley, CA: University of California Press.

Fleury, J. D. (1991). Empowering potential: A theory of wellness motivation. *Nursing Research, 40,* 286–291.

Gallant, R., Cohen, C., & Wolff, T. (1985). Change of older persons' image: Impact on public policy result from Highland Valley empowerment plan. *Perspectives on Aging, 14*(5), 9–13.

Germain, C. (1986). Ethnography: The method. In P. L. Munhall, & C. J. Oiler, (Eds.) *Nursing research: A qualitative perspective*, (pp. 147–162). Norwalk, CT: Appleton-Century-Crofts.

Gibson, C. H. (1991). A concept analysis of empowerment. *Journal of Advanced Nursing, 16,* 354–361.

Gruber, J., & Trickett, E. J. (1987). Can we empower others?: A paradox of empowerment in governing of an alternative public school. *American Journal of Community Psychology, 15,* 353–371.

Haney, P. (1988). Providing empowerment to the person with AIDS. *Social Work, 33,* 251–253.

Hasenfeld, Y., & Cheser, M. A. (1989). Client empowerment in the human services: Personal and professional agenda. *Journal of Applied Behavioral Science, 25,* 499–521.

Ingram, R. (1988). Empower. *Social Policy, 19*(2), 11–16.

Johnstone, M. (1989). Professional ethics and patient's rights: Past realities, future imperatives. *Nursing Forum, 14*(3), 29–34.

Joyce, B., Staley, D., & Hughes, L. (1990). Staying well: Factors contributing to successful community adaptation. *Journal of Psychosocial Nursing, 28*(6), p. 19–24.

Kieffer, C. H. (1984). Citizen empowerment: A developmental perspective. *Prevention in Human Services, 3,* 9–35.

Labonte, R. (1989). Community and professional empowerment. *Canadian Nurse, 85*(3), 23–28.

Langer, E. J., & Rodin, J. (1976). The effects of choice and enhanced personal responsibility for the aged: A field experiment in an institutional setting. *Journal of Personality and Social Psychology, 34,* 191–198.

Leininger, M. M. (1985). *Qualitative research methods in nursing.* Orlando, FL: Grune & Stratton, Inc.

Lincoln, Y. S., & Guha, E. G. (1985). *Naturalistic inquiry.* Beverly Hills, CA: Sage Publications.

Maag, J. (1991). Merriam 'drop-in center' a boon to mental health clients. *The Journal Herald,* n.d.

Malin, N., & Teasdale, K. (1991). Caring versus empowerment: Considerations for nursing practice. *Journal of Advanced Nursing, 16,* 657–662.

Mason, D. J., Costello-Nickitas, D. M., Scanlan, J. M., & Magnuson, B. A. (1991). Empowering nurses for politically astute change in the workplace. *Journal of Continuing Education, 22,* 5–10.

Maton, K. I., & Rappaport, J. (1984). Empowerment in a religious setting: A multivariate investigation. *Prevention in Human Services, 3*(2/3), 37–71.

McMurray, A. (1991). Advocacy for community self-empowerment. *International Nursing Review, 38*(1), 19–21.

Mental Health Amendments of 1990. Public Law 101–639. Title V. (1990).

Minkler, M., & Cox, K. (1980). Creating critical consciousness in health: Applications of Freire's philosophy and methods to the health care setting. *International Journal of Health Services, 10,* 311–322.

Morrissey, J. P., & Goldman, H. H. (1984). Cycles of reform in the care of the chronically mentally ill. *Hospital and Community Psychiatry, 35,* 785–793.

Morten, A., Kohl, M., O'Mahoney, P., & Pelosi, K. (1991). Certified nurse-midwifery care of the postpartum client: A descriptive study. *Journal of Nurse-Midwifery, 36,* 276–284.

Moxley, D. P., & Freddolino, P. P. (1990). A model of advocacy for promoting client self-determination in psychosocial rehabilitation. *Psychosocial Rehabilitation Journal, 14*(2), 69–82.

O'Sullivan, M. J., Waugh, N., & Espeland, W. (1984). The Fort McDowell Yavapai: From pawns to powerbrokers. *Prevention in Human Services, 3*(2/3), 37–71.

Parker, B., & McFarlane, J. (1991). Feminist theory and nursing: An empowerment model for research. *Advances in Nursing Science, 13*(3), 59–67.

Rappaport, J. (1984). Studies in empowerment: Introduction to the issue. *Prevention in Human Services, 3*(2/3), 1–7.

Rappaport, J., Seidman, E., Toro, P. A., McFadden, L. S., Reischl, T. M., Roberts, L. J., et al. (1985). Collaborative research with a mutual help organization. *Social Policy,* Winter, 12–24.

Spradley, J. P. (1979). *The ethnographic interview.* Fort Worth, TX: Holt, Rinehart & Winston.

Spradley, J. P., & McCurdy, D. M. (1972). T*he cultural experience: Ethnography in complex society,* Chicago, IL: Science Research Associates, Inc.

State Comprehensive Mental Health Act of 1986. Public Law 99-660, Title V. (1986).

Tobias, M. (1990). Validator: A key role in empowering the chronically mentally ill. *Social Work, 35,* 357–359.

Wallerstein, N. (1992). Powerlessness, empowerment, and health: Implications for health promotion programs. *American Journal of Health Promotion, 6,* 197–205.

Zinman, S. (1982). A patient-run residence. *Psychosocial Rehabilitation Journal, 6*(1), 3–11.

Lynne M. Connelly, RN, MS, Delta, is LTC (U.S. Army) and a doctoral student, University of Kansas School of Nursing. Becky S. Keele, RN, MS, Gamma Upsilon, Susan V.M. Kleinbeck, RN, MS, Epsilon Gamma, and Joanne Kraenzle Schneider, RN, MN, Epsilon Gamma, are doctoral students at the University of Kansas School of Nursing. Ann Kuckelrnan Cobb, RN, PhD, is Professor at the same institution. The views expressed in this article are those of the authors and do not reflect official policy or position of the Department of the Army, Department of Defense or the U.S. Government. Correspondence to LTC Connelly, University of Kansas School of Nursing, 3901 Rainbow Boulevard, Kansas City, KS 66160-7501.

Accepted for publication November 6, 1992.

CHAPTER 7

Now It Is Your Turn to Analyze Research

As I mentioned earlier, the more practice you have analyzing and critiquing research studies, the easier it will become. In Chapter 6, I presented critiques of two quantitative and two qualitative studies. Now, it is time for you to take a stab at it. The first article that we will start with is a qualitative study about teenage pregnancy. I will only present excerpts from the study here, but you can retrieve a full text copy of the article using the following reference and a database such as CINAHL. Examples of some of the more common databases were presented in Chapter 2. The full reference: Spear, H. (2001). Teenage pregnancy: "Having a baby won't affect me that much." *Pediatric Nursing*, *27*, 574–580. The second article we will use can be found using the following reference: Kunert, K., King, M., & Kolkhost, F. (2007). Fatigue and sleep quality in nurses. *Journal of Psychosocial Nursing*, *45*, 31–37. I will be providing even less information from this article and only the answers to the critique questions first presented in Chapter 6. I would suggest that you take the 10 steps from Table 6-1 and Table 6-2 and a copy of the article and try to do your own critique before reading mine. Okay, time to dive in!

QUALITATIVE RESEARCH STUDY EXAMPLE USING THE TEN STEPS

Problem Study Was Designed to Solve

What is the problem the study was conducted to resolve?

The problem this study was designed to solve can be found in the beginning sentences of this article: sexual activity in adolescence and teen pregnancy that can result from this activity. Spear (2001) goes on to make the argument that "few qualitative studies have examined the experiences and perspectives of young mothers after they have given birth" (p. 574, column 2).

Why is the problem an important one for nursing practice?

The problem is significant for nursing practice in that insight into the daily experience of pregnancy from a teen's perspective can provide the basis for developing appropriate nursing interventions (p. 575, column 1). **(Score: 5)**

Research Question(s)/Hypothesis(es)

What is the purpose of the study?

The purpose of the study is to "gain insight into the day-to-day experience of pregnancy from the perspectives of pregnant adolescents as a basis for developing appropriate nursing interventions to promote their physical and psychological health and socioeconomic well being" (p. 575, column 1, right before the method heading).

What rationale do the authors give to support a qualitative approach?

The author gives clear rationale for using a qualitative design. The first sentence under the methods states, "A naturalistic, qualitative design was selected because it allows for open discovery and documentation of participants' personal perspectives and views" (p. 575, column 1).

What is the research question? If it is not stated, what would you say the research question is?

The author did not state a specific research question; however, the purpose statement can be easily transformed into a research question. For example, the research question could be, "What is the day-to-day experience of pregnancy for a group of adolescents?"

Would you say that the question is stated broadly enough for a qualitative study?

This question is broad enough to allow a variety of data to be collected. **(Score: 3/5)**

Literature Review/Study Framework

Does the particular qualitative method selected call for a literature review and/or conceptual framework prior to initiating fieldwork?

No specific qualitative method was identified, only that the design was naturalistic and qualitative. However, the characteristics of the study design match very well with phenomenology. Looking at the subjective experience of how pregnancy is experienced by these teens by identifying themes, participant's stories, and cases are all characteristics of a phenomenological framework. As with most qualitative methods, only a small amount of literature review was done prior to the fieldwork. Literature presented focused on providing the reader with rationale for why this study was undertaken. Rates of teen pregnancy and how this issue has been studied in the past was the focus of the review (p. 574).

If so, is the review sufficiently comprehensive?

The review is sufficiently comprehensive in that it provides the reader with a foundation about the problem and prior research on teen pregnancy emphasizing the gaps.

Are major concepts identified and defined?

The major concepts are teen pregnancy and the challenges related to teenage pregnancy and childbearing. The author also makes the argument that to truly understand these challenges and develop effective nursing interventions, we need to understand it from the teen's perspective (p. 575, column 1).

If a literature review is appropriate only after data collection, does the researcher outline a process for accomplishing this?

This author did not describe dictates regarding literature review. Since the author identified no specific methodology, this is not required.

If bracketing assumptions are an important component of the qualitative method selected, is this process explained?

Bracketing was not discussed by this author and may be considered a limitation of the study.

Are the majority of references cited within the last 5 years?

Of the 62 total references, 39 were older than 5 years from publication. However, several of these references were classic works on child development, qualitative methodology, and theory. **(Score: 3/5)**

Study Design

What was the qualitative study design used? If design is not made explicit by the authors, can you easily determine what design is being used? Based on what rationale?

As already mentioned, the study design was qualitative. Even though the researcher does not identify a specific qualitative design, it follows well the characteristics of phenomenology.

In what ways is the design an appropriate one to answer the research question or purpose statement?

The design is an appropriate one since the purpose of the design and the purpose of the study are similar, that is to gain insight into the experience of pregnancy for these adolescents. **(Score: 3/5)**

Sample and Setting

Are the sample's characteristics (demographics, size) appropriate based on design and setting? Rationale for answer?

An alternative school program for pregnant teens ages 13 to 19 years served as the setting for this study. This is an appropriate setting given the purpose of the study. The authors do explain that the only difference between this alternative school program and the traditional school is the availability of onsite day care and the inclusion of childcare education. Eight of the nine girls attending the school at the time of the study volunteered to participate in the study (p. 575, columns 1 and 2). **(Score: 4/5)**

Identification and Control of Extraneous Variables

Any threats to rigor? How are the authors addressing these threats?

The author clearly states the methods that were used to establish credibility of the data. For example, a peer auditor was asked to review the raw data and methodological log. They were also asked to evaluate the coherence and clarity of the researcher's interpretations (p. 575, column 3). Further, a consultant who was an experienced qualitative researcher served as auditor throughout the study (p. 576, top of column 1). **(Score: 5/5)**

Study Instruments

What instruments were used to collect data?

A semi-structured interview guide was used to conduct the interviews. This guide had been reviewed by a child development specialist. Sample prompts were given and interviews were audiotaped. After the initial interviews were completed and transcribed, follow-up interviews were conducted. It would have been helpful if the author had shared some of the questions from the interview guide.

Appropriateness of these instruments based on study design?

Interviews using human as instrument is a common method to collect data in qualitative research methodologies. **(Score: 3/5)**

Data Collection Methods

In what ways were the data collection procedures appropriate for the study?

Participants were interviewed individually in a private room at the school during the course of the school day. The initial interview took approximately 1 hour to complete and was done in a conversational style. The second interview took approximately 40 minutes and was used to address areas of interest identified in the first interview. One concern that the researcher mentioned was possible contamination between participants since there was a strong possibility that the participants discussed their interviews with each other (p. 575, columns 2 and 3).

In what ways were appropriate steps taken to protect the rights of study participants? Who approved the study?

Written informed consent was obtained from each participant and her parent or guardian. Approvals and permission to conduct the study were obtained from the university Institutional Review Board and the school board and administration respectively (p. 575, column 2).

Does the researcher outline a plan for keeping data organized and retrievable? Explain your answer.

This was not addressed by this researcher. **(Score: 3/5)**

Data Analysis Procedures

In what ways were the data analysis procedures appropriate for the data collected?

The data analysis was appropriate for the data since the data consisted of word-for-word narratives from the interviews. The analysis began with data reduction by identifying major story lines as supported by Sandelowski, Holditch-Davis, and Harris (1992). Data reduction resulted in the development of individual narrative cases or texts that were then submitted to hermeneutic analysis. By this analysis, data was further reduced to categories and then to themes (p. 575, column 3).

Did the data analysis match the study design? Why or why not?

The data analysis did match the qualitative approach identified by this researcher. However, it would have been better if the researcher had also identified a specific qualitative design rather than just a general qualitative approach.

What evidence is there that data saturation was achieved?

The author explicitly answered this question with the following statement: "Data saturation occurred by the eighth initial interview; conversations were almost predictable at that point (p.575, column 2)." **(Score: 4)**

Overall Findings/Strengths/Limitations

What were the main findings?

Overall, participants expressed a sense of optimism and confidence in their abilities to handle the challenges of parenthood. One of the other major findings was that 75 of the participants indicated that they had physically fought with other females before getting pregnant. The author translated this behavior into the possibility of limited coping skills and immature social interactions with others. The author makes the argument that comprehensive support services need to be available to these individuals for any long-term success (finishing school, attending college, fewer subsequent pregnancies) (pp. 578–579).

What were the major strengths of the study?

- Establishment of credibility of the data
- Data saturation
- Study helped to fill gap in research over the topic from the participant's perspective

What were the major limitations of the study?

- Participants most likely discussed the interviews with each other
- Conducted over a short time period (16 weeks)
- One very specific setting where the participants were already receiving support and resources

Lack of specific qualitative research design identified **(Score: 3/5)**

Total Score: 36 (Fair)

Well, how did you do? By now, it should be coming easier for you. If not, I would suggest going back through Chapter 4 and repeating the steps again. Now, let's move forward with the second article, which is a quantitative research study. It can be found using the following reference: Kunert, K., King, M., & Kolkhost, F. (2007). Fatigue and sleep quality in nurses. *Journal of Psychosocial Nursing, 45*, 31–37. The following sections outline an example of how this article could be critiqued.

QUANTITATIVE RESEARCH STUDY EXAMPLE USING THE TEN STEPS

Problem Statement

What is the problem the study was conducted to resolve?

The problem statement is that fatigue has been shown to be a factor in medical errors and that little is known about the comparison of fatigue and sleep quality between night shift and day shift nurses. The problem was clearly identified by the title of the article and the opening paragraphs.

Why is the problem an important one for nursing practice?

Significance to nursing is highlighted by the authors in the opening paragraphs: "Fatigue is a critical issue for nurses because it cascades to other undesirable outcomes, such as medication errors, degradation in performance, decreased mental acuity, personal problems ..." (abstract and p. 32, column 1). **(Score: 5)**

Research Question(s)/Hypothesis(es)/Study Variables

What are the research questions and/or hypothesis statements?

There were no specific research questions or hypothesis statements found in the article. However, since this is a descriptive design, it is common to have only a purpose statement. The purpose statement was "to examine the differences in perceptions of fatigue between night-shift and day-shift nurses, as measured by scores on the Brief Fatigue Inventory (BFI) and to examine the differences in sleep quality between the two groups, as measured by responses on the Pittsburgh Sleep Quality Index (PSQI)" (p. 32. column 1). Creating a research question and hypothesis statements from the purpose statement can be done easily. For example, a research question could be, "What are the differences in perceptions of fatigue between night-shift and day-shift nurses?"and, "What are the differences in sleep quality between the two groups?" One of the hypothesis statements could be "Night-shift nurses will report more fatigue and less quality of sleep than day-shift nurses."

What are the study variables (both independent and dependent)?

The independent variable here would be the shift the nurse worked, and the dependent variables would be level of fatigue and sleep quality. **(Score: 4.5)**

Literature Review/Background/Framework

Is the literature review sufficient to understand the problem of the study? Can you find a theoretical framework? If so, what is it?

The literature review was sufficient for understanding the problem. Several references on the relationship between fatigue and sleep quality and medical errors were presented. Much of the background consisted of explaining the relationship of fatigue and poor sleep quality to circadian rhythm and the sleep-wake cycle (p. 32, column 2). This was the theoretical framework for the study. The authors present support for this study by discussing how night-shift workers must fight this "body clock" phenomenon to stay awake while at work, particularly between 3 and 5 a.m. They also discuss that night-shift workers tend to experience lighter, shorter, and more fragmented sleep than nighttime sleepers (p. 32, columns 2 and 3; p. 33, column 1).

Are the majority of references cited within the last 5 years?

The majority of the references cited were within the last 5 years of publication date with 18 out of 24 total references dated 2002 or more recently. **(Score: 4.5)**

Study Design/Sample/Setting

What was the quantitative study design used? In what ways is the design an appropriate one to answer the research question/hypothesis/problem statement?

The study used a descriptive design (p. 33, column 2). I think the design should have at least been called a comparative descriptive design since they are comparing two groups (day-shift versus night-shift nurses) on sleep quality and fatigue.

Any threats to internal and external validity? How are the authors addressing these threats?

Threats to validity were not discussed. However, due to the lack of rigor in descriptive level research and the fact that only one hospital was sampled, generalizability of findings (external validity) is limited.

Is the sample appropriate based on design and setting and representativeness of the population? What rationale was used to support sample size (e.g., power analysis)?

The sample was a convenience sample of 90 night-shift and 100 day-shift nurses. Based on a power analysis using 0.8 power, alpha of 0.05 and a moderate effect size of 0.4, 98 night-shift and 98 day-shift nurses would be required

(p. 33, column 2). The sample did not include the required amount of night-shift nurses. However, the statistical analyses were significant with the night shift scoring higher on both the fatigue and sleep quality indices. Therefore, the effect size was large enough to detect differences even with a smaller number in the night-shift group. **(Score: 3.5)**

Identification and Control of Extraneous Variables

What are the main extraneous variables? What ways are the authors controlling for them?

Extraneous variables were not explicitly identified by the authors in this study. However, they did statistically examine the effects of several variables that could have been potential extraneous variables. For example, age of the nurse and work experience could have been potential extraneous variables. Night-shift nurses had higher fatigue and PSQI scores than day-shift nurses. Night-shift nurses were younger and had less nursing experience than day-shift nurses. **(Score: 3)**

Study Instruments

What were the instruments (both physiologic and psychological) used to collect data for the study? What validity and reliability measures were reported for each? Were the selected instruments adequate to measure the study's variables? Why or why not?

Two primary instruments were used in the study; the Brief Fatigue Inventory (BFI) and the Pittsburgh Sleep Quality Index (PSQI). For the BFI, validity and reliability for this study was reported with a Cronbach's alpha of 0.91 and a one-factor solution factor analysis accounting for 76% of the total variance. For the PSQI, Cronbach's alpha was 0.71 for this study. Factor analysis resulted in three factors accounting for 40%, 17%, and 14% of the variance respectively (p. 33, columns 2 and 3; p. 34, column 1). The instruments were adequate since they were designed to measure the variables of interest in the study: fatigue and sleep quality. **(Score: 4.5)**

Data Collection Methods

In what ways were the data collection procedures appropriate for the study? In what ways were appropriate steps taken to protect the rights of study participants? Who approved the study? How did the data collection methods match the study design?

Study was approved by the institutional review board (p. 33, column 1). Nurses were sampled from the medical–surgical, intensive care, telemetry, surgery, emergency, and recovery units (p. 33, column 2). A cover letter explaining the study, along with a consent form and the BFI and the PSQI, were distributed to the nurses' unit mailboxes. Return rate was very high at 96% (p. 34, column 1). **(Score: 5)**

Data Analysis Procedures

In what ways were the data analysis procedures appropriate for the data collected? Did the data analysis match the study design? Why or why not?

Descriptive statistics were used to examine categorical data such as demographic data (p. 34, column 1). Univariate analysis was used to test the mean differences in scores between the day-shift and night-shift nurses on the total BFI and global PSQI scores. Multivariate analysis was used to test mean differences on subscale scores on the PSQI between the two groups. Regression analysis was used to determine which PSQI subscales predicted fatigue (p. 34, column 1 and 2). It is interesting to note that the authors did not give the specific univariate or multivariate analyses conducted. This would have been helpful to discern whether or not the correct specific statistical test had been chosen. **(Score: 3.5)**

Overall Findings/Strengths/Limitations

What were the main findings?

The night-shift nurses had overall poorer sleep quality than the day-shift nurses with significant differences found both on the BFI and the PSQI. Demographically, nurses with more years of experience and either married or divorced reported greater levels of fatigue and poorer sleep quality than nurses with less experience and who were single. Predictors of fatigue in night-shift nurses were sleep medication use and daytime dysfunction (p. 35, columns 1, 2, and 3; p. 36, columns 1 and 2).

What were the major strengths of the study? What were the major limitations of the study?

Several strengths and limitations can be discerned from this article. Many of the study's findings supported prior research findings over the same issue. However, this study added to prior work by finding that day-shift nurses also used medication to help them sleep after shift work. Strong implications for nursing were suggested as the result of this study's findings. For example, nurses should be encouraged to take regularly scheduled breaks including meal breaks and avoid overtime. Promoting physical activity and providing resources to do so was another strong recommendation by these authors to increase energy, sleep quality, and fitness of nurses and to reduce fatigue.

Another interesting suggestion was to encourage organizations to develop napping policies and encourage short scheduled naps by nurses particularly on the night shift (p. 36, columns 2 and 3).

The authors did a good job of describing the instruments used in the study and reporting validity and reliability measures, particularly for their study. Fatigue and poor sleep quality are significant issues for nurses doing shift work, and recommendations from the findings of this study provide some feasible strategies to implement in the workplace.

Since several prior research studies had already been done on this issue, it would have been better if the authors had selected a stronger research design rather than just a descriptive study. Possibly a correlational study would have been a better choice and would have provided stronger findings. Along the same lines, selecting a random sample would have increased the validity of the study's findings (p. 36, column 3). Since both day-shift and night-shift nurses experienced fatigue and lack of sleep quality, it would be interesting in future work to examine length of shift as a possible culprit for these findings since both groups were working 12-hour shifts. **(Score: 4)**

Total Score: 42.5 (Good)

Whew! I bet you are getting the knack of doing research article critiques by now! If not, I would suggest going back to Chapter 6 and the beginning of this chapter at least one more time through with the examples provided. If you are feeling comfortable enough to move on, we will do just two more articles. This time I will provide the reference and examples of how this article could be critiqued but without reference as to where the answers can be found within the article. I am also only providing the 10 steps to critiquing quantitative nursing research studies. See Table 6-1 and Table 6-2 if you need a review of the specific questions to ask within each step. Are you ready? Okay, let's go!

The first article is a qualitative study exploring midlife women's attitudes toward physical activity. You can search and find this article with the following reference: Im, E., Chee, W., Lim, H., Liu, Y., & Kim, H. (2008). Midlife women's attitudes toward physical activity. *JOGNN, 37,* 203–213. Now that you have a full text copy of this article in front of you, we will begin by taking the same 10 steps we have already been using with other qualitative research studies. To begin with, the title often gives the reader a hint about what research methodology was used. In this case, the researchers are looking at attitudes, and qualitative research provides a great forum to elicit not only the attitudes but the meaning behind these attitudes. Another place to find hints about the type of study that was done is by looking at the abstract. From the abstract, we find that the design used was a qualitative cross-sectional study using an online forum. Now that we have figured out that this is a qualitative study, it is time to take the 10 steps for critiquing qualitative nursing research articles.

QUALITATIVE STUDY EXAMPLE FOR YOU TO DO ON YOUR OWN

Problem the Study Was Designed to Solve

The authors do a good job of presenting the problem this study was designed to solve. The problem is lack of physical activity for ethnic midlife women. Further, they go on to make the argument that despite the number of studies on physical activity, little is known about ethnic midlife women's attitudes toward physical activity. Even though the authors do not explicitly state why the problem is important for nursing practice, they do present the potential negative health effects of lack of physical activity. They also discuss how important it is to incorporate women's attitudes toward physical activity into promotion interventions. **(Score: 4)**

Purpose Statement/Research Question(s)

The purpose statement was difficult to find within the narrative of the article. I think part of the problem was the fact that the study had three sections: Internet survey, expert interview, and online forum, with only the online forum findings being presented. However, it was easy to find within the abstract of the article, "to explore attitudes toward physical activity among a multiethnic group of midlife women." The rationale for using a qualitative approach was not clear. However, the authors do state that little is known about midlife women's attitudes toward physical activity. As discussed in earlier chapters, when little is known about a problem, qualitative research is a very appropriate method to explore the problem and issues surrounding the problem. The research question was not stated; however, the purpose statement can be easily developed into a question. The research question could be "What are the attitudes toward physical activity among a multiethnic group of midlife women?" This is definitely broad enough to explore as a qualitative study. **(Score: 2)**

Literature Review/Study Framework

It is hard to know if a literature review/conceptual framework is needed before fieldwork for this study since the authors did not identify a specific qualitative method. A fairly comprehensive literature review was presented, and the conceptual framework of feminism was applied in the study. Fifty-two references were included in the beginning literature review, with 17 references over 5 years old from the date of this publication. Major concepts were defined very well. For example, attitudes toward physical activity were defined as "what a woman thinks and expresses about a physically active lifestyle for herself." Bracketing is not discussed at all in this study. **(Score: 3)**

Study Design

The only place that the design was clearly stated was in the abstract. In the abstract the authors state that the design was a qualitative cross-sectional study using an online forum. They do not state any particular qualitative methodology. The authors discuss a thematic analysis, which could be interpreted as a phenomenology, but this is not stated. Qualitative methods were appropriate to use in this study since the purpose was to explore attitudes toward physical activity among a multiethnic group of midlife women. **(Score: 2)**

Sample and Setting

The final sample size was 15 participants. The authors provide rationale for the sample being an adequate sample by providing a reference that supports 6 to 10 participants being adequate for a qualitative focus group, including online forums. **(Score: 4)**

Identification and Control for Threats to Rigor

The authors do a good job of explaining how they adhered to standards of rigor in feminist qualitative research including dependability, reflexivity, credibility, relevance, and adequacy. For example, dependability was supported by examining the methodological and analytic decision trails created by the researchers during the study. They go on to explain how they ensured each standard of rigor in the ensuing paragraph. **(Score: 4.5)**

Instruments Used to Collect Data

An online Internet survey was used to collect the data. The authors present the 10 online forum topics on attitudes toward physical activity and 7 online forum topics on ethnic-specific contexts that were used. They did not discuss how they developed these topics. Examples of prompts that were used for one of the online topics (meaning of physical activity to the women) were provided to the reader. The topics are appropriate given the study's purpose and qualitative approach. **(Score: 4)**

Data Collection Methods

A website conforming to Health Insurance Portability and Accountability Act, SysAdmin, Audit, Network, and Security Institute/Federal Bureau of Investigation recommendations was published on an independent website server. The website contained a consent form and explanation of the purpose of the study.

If the participant signed the consent form electronically, then the website queried them about inclusion criteria. If they met the inclusion criteria, they were connected to the survey page. The study was approved by the internal review board of their institution. The data collection methods matched the study design since the purpose of the online forums was to share participants' attitudes toward physical activity with each other. The authors gave details about how the data was collected and organized. For example, they state, "The data was saved in ASCII files and printed out as transcripts. These transcripts were read and reread for line-by-line coding, which was summarized into a codebook." **(Score: 5)**

Data Analysis Procedures

A thematic analysis was used to analyze the data. Line-by-line coding was done and developed into a code book. Identified codes were inductively analyzed to create categories. Relationships between categories were developed based on mapping links among the categories. An interactive process was used to identify themes common across participants. Demographic information was also examined in light of these responses. A separate research team member was used only for the data analysis to ensure consistency. All three researchers were involved in the categorization process. Data saturation was not discussed. **(Score: 4)**

Overall Findings/Strengths/Limitations

The findings of this study indicated that women across ethnic groups were raised by their parents and society to be physically inactive. Women in the study also shared that they had no time for physical activity because of their multiple roles. Physical environment factors, such as poor weather, also played a role in whether participants would participate in physical activity. The majority of participants shared their desire for a companion when exercising, although white women's reason was for fun, whereas ethnic minorities voiced a need for safety.

Strengths of the study include a multiethnic sample, detailed adherence to standards of rigor in qualitative research and a creative methodology of using online focus group forums. Implications for nurses when promoting physical activity with ethnically diverse women include consideration of the multiple roles these women play, and cultural and environmental factors that influence participation in physical activity. Limitations include the majority of the sample being Caucasian or Hispanic (12 out of 15) and no evidence of data saturation. **(Score: 3)**

Total Score: 35.5 (Fair)

The last article analysis is a quantitative study examining neighborhood characteristics, adherence to walking, and depressive symptoms in midlife African-American women. You can search and find this article with the following reference: Wilbur, J., Zenk, S., Wang, E., Oh, A., McDevitt, J., Block, D., McNeil, S., & Ju, S. (2009). Neighborhood characteristics, adherence to walking, and depressive symptoms in midlife African-American women. *Journal of Women's Health, 18,* 1201–1210. Now, that you have a full text copy of this article in front of you, we can begin by taking the same 10 steps we have already been using with other quantitative research studies. To begin with, the title often gives the reader a hint about what research methodology was used. In this case, the researchers are looking at relationships between neighborhood characteristics and depressive symptoms on adherence to walking. Another place to find hints about the type of study that was done is by looking at the abstract. From the abstract, we find that the design was testing a physical activity intervention and the relationship between adherence to the intervention and depressive symptoms and neighborhood characteristics. However, it is not until the body of the paper that we find that this study actually used a quasi-experimental design. Now, that we have figured out that this is a quantitative study, let's take the 10 steps for critiquing quantitative nursing research articles and get started.

QUANTITATIVE STUDY EXAMPLE FOR YOU TO DO ON YOUR OWN

Problem the Study Was Designed to Solve

The problem is not clearly identified by the authors of this study. After reading the introduction multiple times, it appears that the primary problem is depressive symptoms in African-American women. However, they also discuss the effects of neighborhood characteristics on depressive symptoms in this population. Further, they discuss the relationship of physical activity and depressive symptoms. So, it is difficult to determine the actual problem. Is it depressive symptoms, is it the negative effects of neighborhood characteristics, or is it lack of physical activity of African-American women? The problem is significant to nursing if it is lack of physical activity for this ethnic population. However, since this article was published in a nonnursing journal (*Journal of Women's Health*), its audience is not just nurses but other providers who are interested in women's health. **(Score: 2)**

Research Question(s)/Hypothesis(es)

Hypothesis statements include "At the end of 24 weeks, the enhanced treatment women compared with the minimal treatment women would have greater improvement in their depressive symptoms." They also hypothesized "that controlling for individual characteristics, walking adherence at 24 weeks would be associated with lower depressive symptoms, whereas neighborhood deterioration and crime would be associated with higher depressive symptoms." Lastly, the researchers hypothesized "that walking adherence would moderate the effects of neighborhood deterioration and crime on depressive symptoms at 24 weeks." For the first hypothesis, the independent variable is the enhanced treatment versus minimal treatment, and the dependent variable is depressive symptoms. For the second hypothesis, walking adherence, individual characteristics, neighborhood deterioration, and crime would be the independent variables, and depressive symptoms would be the dependent variable. For the last hypothesis, walking adherence, neighborhood deterioration, and crime would be the independent variables and depressive symptoms would be the dependent variable. **(Score: 5)**

Literature Review/Study Framework

Many of the references cited were older than 5 years from the date of publication (2009). Over half (25 out of 40) of the references used in the introduction/background were older. Other than many of the references being somewhat old, the authors do provide a good foundation of prior research related to neighborhood characteristics, depressive symptoms, and physical activity for African-American women. A theoretical framework is not evident; however, a loosely defined conceptual framework can be identified with difficulty. It appears that the authors are making the connection between the prevalence of depressive symptoms with the African-American women population. They also make the argument that neighborhood characteristics (more hazards and fewer resources) have a direct relationship to depressive symptoms, and that there is an inverse relationship between physical activity and depressive symptoms. It is also noteworthy to mention that behavioral strategies were based on Social Cognitive Theory and the Transtheoretical Model. However, this was not mentioned until the intervention was discussed. **(Score: 2)**

Study Design

A quasi-experimental design was used in this study. To prevent the threat of treatment contamination, the community health centers used in the study were randomly assigned into treatment groups rather than individuals within each center being randomly assigned between the two treatment groups. The samples at each center were of convenience and were not randomly assigned. Other than treatment contamination, no specific threats to validity were discussed. The quasi-experimental design is an appropriate one to answer the research study's hypotheses since the main hypothesis was to compare treatment (enhanced versus minimal). Both groups received a tailored walking prescription, but the enhanced treatment group also received four weekly motivational workshops along with tailored supportive staff telephone calls weekly for 3 weeks. **(Score: 2)**

Sample and Setting

For the most part, the sample is appropriate for the quasi-experimental design used. The main weakness of the sample is that it was not initially selected randomly. However, the two participating community centers were randomized into the two treatment options. No rationale was provided to support the final sample size of 278 women. **(Score: 3)**

Identification and Control of Extraneous Variables

Age, marital status, education, income, and body mass index were identified as potential extraneous variables and were controlled for statistically by using them as covariates in the analyses. **(Score: 5)**

Study Instruments

The 20-item CES-D scale was used to assess depressive symptoms. Internal consistency measured by a Cronbach's alpha was 0.71 for this study, barely above the minimum acceptable level of 0.70. Validity measures were not provided, only a reference. Walking adherence frequency was calculated as the percentage of the prescribed 68 walks. Adherence was measured using heart rate monitors, logbook, and an automated telephone system. No measures of reliability or validity were given. The authors did state that they compared data from these three sources and removed any duplicate data. They also presented in some detail as to how they measured neighborhood characteristics including deterioration and crime. For example, crime was measured as the annual number of police-reported incidents of violent person-to-person crimes in the neighborhood. Perceived neighborhood crime was measured with seven items from the Neighborhood Problems Scale. Description and scoring instructions were provided along with a reference but no specific validity measures were given. Internal consistency reliability was 0.90.

Instruments used were specific to the variables of interest to the researchers (depressive symptoms, walking adherence, and neighborhood characteristics) and are therefore adequate to measure these variables. The main limitation of these measures is the lack of any validity measures reported in this study. **(Score: 3)**

Data Collection Methods

Women were recruited into one of two community health centers: the enhanced treatment or the minimal treatment groups. Social networking, newspaper announcements, and presentations were some of the strategies used to recruit participants. Participants were staggered into the study over 3.5 years. Women in both groups received a tailored walking prescription. Depressive symptoms were measured both at baseline and at the end of the study. It is unclear if the minimal treatment group was treated only individually or if there was encouragement to walk as a group. The four motivational workshops that the enhanced treatment group received were conducted in a group setting. Therefore, this interaction between participants may also provide needed support to facilitate walking adherence and to influence depressive symptoms over and above the workshop content. This was not addressed by the researchers until the end of the study. Steps taken to protect the rights of participants were not addressed and are a weakness of this article. **(Score: 2)**

Data Analysis Procedures

Paired samples T-tests were performed comparing baseline to end of study (24 weeks). This is appropriate given the interval level data obtained from the CES-D scale. Regression was used to examine the effects of the ET on depressive symptoms while controlling for the covariates mentioned earlier. Regression was also used to examine the effects of walking adherence on depressive symptoms. The analyses were appropriate for answering the study's hypotheses and testing the effects of the intervention using a quasi-experimental design. **(Score: 5)**

Overall Findings/Strengths/Limitations

Adjusting for demographics, body mass index, and depressive symptoms at baseline, walking adherence and objective neighborhood deterioration were associated with lower depressive symptoms. Perceived neighborhood characteristics were associated with higher levels of depressive symptoms at the end of the study.

The major strengths of the study included a novel approach to examining the influence of adherence to walking and neighborhood characteristics on depressive symptoms by using a behavioral physical activity intervention, particularly in African-American women. Another strength of this study was the use of two different-sized radial buffers (1 mile and .25 mile) around their homes to define neighborhoods of the participants, which provided a more precise description of the area surrounding the participants' homes.

The authors do a good job of identifying some of the major limitations of the study. They include neighborhoods that were not sampled to assure the best possible variation of neighborhood characteristics, treatments that were randomly assigned to sites rather than women being assigned to treatment conditions, and the inability to tease out the effects of social support gained from being in the enhanced treatment group on depressive symptoms. Other limitations not identified by the authors include lack of clearly stated problem statement, majority of references older than 5 years, lack of a clearly defined and applied theoretical framework, omitted information on the validity of instruments used, and protection of participant rights. **(Score: 4)**

Total Score: 33 (Poor)

THE BIG "SO WHAT?"

- The more practice you have analyzing and critiquing research studies, the easier it will become.
- Results from a research study should only be considered for implementation in nursing practice if the score for rigor is at least 35 (Fair).

REFERENCES

Im, E. O., Chee, W., Lim, H., Liu, Y., & Kim, H. (2008). Midlife women's attitudes toward physical activity. *Journal of Obstetric, Gynecologic, & Neonatal Nursing, 37*, 203–213.

Kunert, K. (2007). Fatigue and sleep quality in nurses. *Journal of Psychosocial Nursing, 45*, 31–37.

Spear, H. (2001). Teenage pregnancy: "Having a baby won't affect me that much." *Pediatric Nursing, 27*, 574–580.

Wilbur, J., Zenk, S., Wang, E., Oh, A., McDevitt, J., Block, D., et al. (2009). Neighborhood characteristics, adherence to walking, and depressive symptoms in midlife African American women. *Journal of Women's Health, 18*, 1201–1210.

CHAPTER 8

Ethics in Research and Evidence-Based Nursing Practice

ETHICS IN NURSING RESEARCH

Ethics Defined

Chaloner (2007) states that "Ethics is a branch of philosophy concerned with determining right and wrong in relation to people's decisions and actions." Ethics is concerned with rules and principles of human behavior. Applied to research, ethical research means that participants' rights are preserved. These rights include freedom from harm; right to withdraw from a study without consequences, to be treated fairly, and to have their identity protected. It is the nurse's responsibility to be informed about the rights of human subjects in nursing research. An examination of some of the most critical historical events influencing research ethics is necessary for understanding measures implemented to protect a human subject's rights in research today.

Historical Events Influencing Ethics in Research

The first international effort to establish formal ethical guidelines for human subject research is the Nuremberg Code, developed in 1947. This was in response to the sadistic experiments performed on Jewish concentration camp prisoners during World War II. One such atrocity was performed on 112 Jewish prisoners in 1944 (Nieswiadomy, 2008). After photographs and body measurements were taken, they were killed and defleshed. One purported purpose of the study was to determine if photographs from live human beings could predict actual skeletal size. The Nuremberg Code requires informed consent in all cases, makes no provision for any special treatment of children, the elderly, or the mentally incompetent, and disallows any research on subjects who are not capable of giving consent.

The Declaration of Helsinki, published in 1964 by the World Medical Association, is a guide for medical doctors engaged in biomedical research. Revised several times, the latest revision occurred during the 52nd World Medical Association General Assembly in Edinburgh, Scotland in 2000. The National Commission for the Protection of Human Subjects of Biomedical and Behavioral Research published a report in 1979 entitled *The Belmont Report*. The Nuremberg Code, Declaration of Helsinki, and the Belmont Report can be found in the IRB Guidebook at http://www.hhs.gov/ohrp/irb/irb_appendices.htm#j7. Three basic principles from the Belmont Report related to human subject research continue to be relevant today:

1. Respect for persons (autonomy and self-determination)
2. Beneficence (do no harm)
3. Justice (fair treatment)

Because of the US Department of Health and Human Services general guidelines for research published in 1981, institutional review boards (IRBs) were created. Every organization or institution that receives federal money for research is required to have IRBs that review research proposals. Along with the IRBs, other research committees that review research proposals include nursing research committees. The Health Insurance Portability and Accountability Act (HIPAA) pertains not only to an individual's health information, but also applies if that health information is used in research. The HIPAA Privacy Rule establishes conditions under which protected health information may be used for research purposes. This rule defines the means by which individuals will be informed of uses and disclosures of their medical information for research purposes, and their rights to access this information. It further protects the privacy of individually identifiable health information, while at the same time ensuring that this type of information is available to conduct needed research. More detail is provided at the US Department of Health and Human Services website: http://privacyruleandresearch.nih.gov/.

Research Guidelines for Nurses

In 1968, the American Nurses Association Research and Studies Commission published their first set of guidelines for nurse researchers. These guidelines have been through several revisions, with the latest being published in 1995. Nine principles that guide nursing research are addressed (Silva, 1995). Not only are human rights addressed, but these guidelines include other areas such as research and cultural diversity, capacity issues, deception in research, scientific integrity and misconduct, use of computers in research, and research with pregnant women, children, or persons with AIDS. The following paragraphs summarize each of these guidelines.

Right to Self-Determine

Persons have the right to choose whether they want to participate in research. This choice should be free from coercion. They also must have the freedom to cease participation at any time. To be able to self-determine, a person must possess decision-making capacity that includes ability to determine a plan of action, comprehend it adequately, and carry out action without undue controlling influences. It is the responsibility of the investigator to assess this capacity prior to and throughout the study. Children that are minors but possess decision-making capacity should be given the choice of assent, along with parental informed consent.

It is critical that the potential research participant be given enough information to make an informed decision about participation. Elements of informed consent include disclosure of needed information, comprehension of this information, competence of the subject to provide consent, and voluntariness of that consent. The information should be free of jargon and written at no higher than a fifth-grade level. Elements normally disclosed in an informed consent are provided in **Table 8-1**.

Strategies to promote comprehension include assessing the reading level required for the written consent form; presenting information in a clear way, using audiovisual aids if needed to help with comprehension; and allowing research participants to review consent forms over several days and discuss with family and friends as needed. Voluntariness is the choice by the person to participate in research without fear of consequences. This includes being able to terminate participation at any time without penalty. Choice to participate should also be free of coercion where the participant participates due to external influences or inducements exerted to the point that the research participant cannot resist. These inducements may involve monetary benefit or other incentives or fear of harm if they do not participate. See **Table 8-2** for a typical consent form and **Table 8-3** for a simplified version of a consent form. Each is appropriate depending on the literacy level expected of the research participants.

Right to Protection from Harm

This principle includes doing no harm (nonmaleficence) and doing good (beneficence). "Doing no harm" is one of the cornerstones of ethical practice. However, there are circumstances that make it necessary to cause risk of some degree of harm to research participants for the greater good. The investigator must weigh potential benefits against potential risks. The greater the risk taken, the greater the benefits should be to the participants. It is the researcher's responsibility to have checks and balances in place and a procedure for handling any negative effects from the research. Silva addresses several

---

Table 8-1   Elements of an Informed Consent

---

1. Subject willingness to participate in a research study
2. Purposes of the study
3. Time commitment
4. Nature of the participation such as number of contacts with the investigator(s) and treatments
5. Expected benefits
6. Alternative procedures or treatments
7. Risks or discomforts that may occur and protocol that will be followed if harm occurs
8. Right to voluntary participation and withdrawal at any time during participation without penalty
9. Protection of anonymity or if not possible, how and under what conditions their identity will be revealed
10. Data security
11. Who is conducting the study and contact persons and information if questions arise
12. Review boards that have examined the study
13. That the research participant's signature on a consent form indicates willingness to participate
14. A witness's signature on a consent form verifies that the person giving consent is who they claim to be

Excerpted from Silva (1995). *Ethical guidelines in the conduct, dissemination, and implementation of nursing research.* Washington, DC: American Nurses Association.

---

vulnerable populations within this ethical principle including children, pregnant women, persons with AIDS, and the elderly.

Respect for Diversity

The investigator should respect the diversity of research participants. All forms of diversity are included, such as age, gender, life style, sexual orientation, and culture. Strategies to ensure culturally competent nursing research include using study instruments that are valid and reliable for that culture, using translators that are not culturally biased, and ensuring research questions/ hypotheses do not promote ethnocentrism.

Table 8-2   Sample Consent Form

PROJECT TITLE: Assessment of Environmental Contaminants on Residents of New Mexico

RESEARCHER
Jane Doe, Ph.D.
Assistant Professor, Department of Biology
New Mexico State University
(575) 646-XXXX

DESCRIPTION
Jane Doe, my colleagues, John Smith, Ph.D. and Jane Jones, Ph.D., and I are members of the Department of Biology at New Mexico State University. We are interested in collecting information on the exposure to environmental pollution of residents of New Mexico. The purpose of this research study is to collect blood, hair, urine, and indoor and outdoor air for analysis of environmental contaminants, including lead, mercury, volatile organic chemicals, and general air quality. It will be necessary to analyze the samples from approximately 300 participants to determine whether there are any health effects related to environmental pollution.

You are being asked to participate in the study because you are a resident of New Mexico. If you decide to participate, you will be asked to visit the Southside Health Clinic on three occasions over a 6-month period, where you will be asked to provide a urine sample, a hair sample, and a blood sample (approximately 30 drops). The hair, urine, and blood will be tested only for the presence of the above-named environmental contaminants. Prior to the first appointment at the clinic, you will fill out a 40-item questionnaire and will be interviewed by one of the above researchers. This will take approximately 1 hour. The appointments at the Southside Health Clinic will take approximately 30 minutes to complete. At the end of the 6-month period, you will be interviewed again by one of the above researchers. This interview will take approximately 1 hour. In addition to the appointments at the Southside Health Clinic, a device that monitors air quality will be installed in your residence for the same 6-month period. This device is approximately the size of a 1 ft square box and is silent. If you decide to participate, you will be paid $50 for each completed appointment at the Southside Health Clinic. Additionally, at the end of the 6-month period, you will receive $50 for agreeing to the installation of the air quality device in your residence. The total compensation will not exceed $200.

EXCLUSION CRITERIA
Participation in the study is restricted to those individuals who have been residents of New Mexico for at least 2 years.

RISKS AND BENEFITS
Obtaining a blood sample can result in a small bruise at the site of the needle insertion, which will usually disappear in 7–14 days, as well as mild discomfort at the time the blood sample is obtained. The hair, urine, and blood will be tested only

(continued)

Table 8-2   Sample Consent Form *(continued)*

for the presence of the above-named environmental contaminants. The research
team will be working with the clinical staff at the Southside Health Clinic, and their
trained professional staff will be assisting in the collection of the samples. The
results of the analyses of hair, urine, blood, and air will be given to you and your
healthcare provider, along with a written explanation. Any needed treatment and
follow-up will be arranged promptly. However, NMSU is not responsible for the cost
of any follow-up treatment. The results of this study may benefit residents of New
Mexico by pointing to the need to reduce the amount of environmental pollutants.

VOLUNTARY NATURE OF PARTICIPATION
You may withdraw from the research study at any time since your participation is
entirely voluntary. If you decide not to participate, there will be no penalty or loss
of benefits to you to which you are otherwise entitled. If you decide to participate,
you may discontinue at a later date without penalty or loss of benefits to you to
which you are otherwise entitled.

CONFIDENTIALITY
Any information obtained about you from the research, including answers to
questionnaires, history, laboratory data findings, or physical examination, will
be kept strictly confidential. The information you give us will not be shared with
anyone outside the research team with your name attached. We will protect your
confidentiality by coding your information with a number so no one can trace
your answers to your name, limiting access to identifiable information, telling the
research staff the importance of confidentiality, and storing research records in
locked cabinets that are accessible only to the three named researchers above.
The data derived from this study could be used in reports, presentations, and
publications, but you will never be individually identified.

NEW INFORMATION
Any new information obtained during the course of the research that may affect
your willingness to continue participation in the study will be provided to you.

SIGNATURE
Your signature below means that you have freely agreed to participate in this
research study. You should consent only if you have read the previous or it has been
read to you and you understand its contents. If you have any questions pertaining
to the research, you may contact the principal investigator, Jane Doe, whose phone
number is (505) 646-XXXX. If you have any questions about your rights as a research
subject, please contact the Institutional Review Board (IRB) chair, through the
Office of Compliance at New Mexico State University at (505) 646-7177 or at
ovpr@nmsu.edu.

Signature _____

Date _____

A copy of this consent form will be given to you to keep.

Excerpted from http://research.nmsu.edu/compliance/IRB/forms.html

Table 8-3 Simplified Sample Consent Form

EXAMINING DIET AND FITNESS AMONG ADOLESCENTS
My name is Mary Smith. I am a professor (teacher) in the Department of Health Sciences at New Mexico State University.

I am asking you to take part in a research study because I am trying to learn more about exercise and nutrition. I want to learn about the types of exercises kids your age do and what kinds of food they eat. Your parent(s) have given you permission to participate in this study.

If you agree, you will be asked to complete a survey (written set of questions). You will be asked how often you exercise and what kind of exercises you do. You will also be asked the kind of foods you eat. You will be asked to provide your height and weight. Answering these questions will take about 15 minutes. You do not have to put your name on the survey. You do not have to answer any questions that make you uncomfortable.

You do not have to be in this study. No one will be mad at you if you decide not to do this study. Even if you start the study, you can stop later if you want. You may ask questions about the study at any time. I will answer any questions you may want to ask.

If you decide to be in the study I will not tell anyone else how you respond or act as part of the study. Even if your parents or teachers ask, I will not tell them about what you say or do in the study.

If you or your child has questions about your rights or those of your child, you can call the Office of the Vice President for Research at (575) 646-7177.

Signing here means that you have read this form, or have had it read to you and that you are willing to be in this study.

Signature of Subject _____

Subject's Printed Name _____

Signature of Investigator _____

Date _____

Excerpted from http://research.nmsu.edu/compliance/IRB/forms.html

Right to Fair Treatment

Some of the most serious violations of human rights have occurred during the selection of research subjects. Historically, two highly publicized studies, the Willowbrook and Tuskegee studies, went on for a long time before they were questioned, deemed unethical, and stopped. The Tuskegee Syphilis Study is a prime example of how this principal can be violated. Research subjects were recruited from a poor area of Macon County, Alabama. The total sample consisted of black sharecroppers who were easy to keep isolated and uninformed as to the purpose of the research. This study is discussed in more detail later in this chapter. This group suffered an unfair disadvantage regarding study burdens and risks.

Right of Privacy, Confidentiality, and Anonymity

Privacy in research is the respect for a participant's willingness to share or refuse to share personal information. Confidentiality and anonymity refer to how others handle private information. The investigator respects the participant's choice on who can have access to their confidential information. This also involves keeping the participant's information secure from people who should not have access. Abiding by this guideline can be complex, particularly in today's research environment with computerization and ability to store large amounts of personal data.

Ethical Integrity of the Research Process

Integrity of the research process is important from its conception through implementation of study findings. If at any point of the process the research is compromised, then the credibility of the whole study is compromised. As proposed in ANA guidelines (Silva, 1995), checks and balances to promote scientific integrity include educational programs, institutional policies and procedures, governmental policies and procedures, peer reviews, and responsible whistle-blowing. Guidelines for authors and editors in publishing findings from nursing research studies are also addressed by these guidelines.

Responsibility to Report Scientific Misconduct

Scientific misconduct is the intentional misrepresentation of any aspect of the research process (Silva, 1995). Examples of misrepresentation include fabrication of data, plagiarism, and any other questionable research practice. The Office of Research Integrity is responsible for overseeing investigations of scientific misconduct. Many funding agencies have also addressed scientific misconduct in grant application materials.

A Competent Investigator

The investigator must maintain competency in the subject matter and methodologies of their research, as well as societal and other issues that affect nursing research and the public (Silva, 1995). Research cannot be performed in isolation from the nursing profession or the larger society as a whole. It is the investigator's responsibility to be knowledgeable about all aspects of the research process. They should also stay informed of any societal factors that might influence the conduct and implementation of research. Human subjects training is available at the National Institutes of Health website: http://phrp. nihtraining.com/users/login.php. Other resources available regarding informed consent and responsible conduct of research can be found at http://bioethics. od.nih.gov/casestudies.html.

Safe Animal Research

As Silva (1995) shares, few nurse investigators are currently prepared for experimentations with animals, which significantly reduces the contributions that can be made to nursing practice. Resources should be made available so that nurse investigators can participate in this type of research. Knowledge and education on the proper care of animal subjects is critical for ethical research using animal subjects.

Case Study of Ethical Violations

One of the most infamous violations of human subjects' rights came not at the hands of some supremacist group such as the Nazis but at the hands of the United States government through the United States Public Health Service (USPHS). Known as the Tuskegee Syphilis Study, it resulted in research abuses of 399 African-American male sharecroppers in Macon County, Alabama. The USPHS wanted to study the effects of untreated syphilis in the black male. The study included 201 subjects without syphilis as controls. Subjects with diagnosed syphilis were given no treatment even though they were promised a special treatment for "bad blood" (Strait, 1993). Subjects received vitamins at best, and the special treatment was a diagnostic painful spinal tap. Subjects were harmed by withholding treatment and being exposed to painful, risky diagnostic procedures. Subjects were coerced into participating by promised treatment for their "bad blood" and enough money to bury them. The USPHS did not disclose all of the facts regarding the study. In fact, the subjects had no idea they were to become research subjects. They just thought they were being treated for their disease. Rights to privacy, confidentiality, and anonymity were violated. Even if the men sought out treatment from other healthcare providers on their own, they were tracked down and not allowed to receive any kind of care. In at least one situation, a physician was reprimanded by the government and the American Medical Association for attempting to provide care to one of the participants. Treatment was nonexistent for these men. Starting in 1932, the study documented at least 28 deaths by 1969 from complications of late-stage syphilis. In July 1972, 40 years after the study started, Jean Heller of the Associated Press broke the story, and the study was stopped (Strait, 1993).

The legacy of such atrocities continues to impact participation in research today. Studies have reported the greater reluctance of African Americans to participate in clinical research studies (Reverby, 2000). However, more recent research (Katz et al., 2009), reports that it is unlikely that detailed knowledge of the Tuskegee Syphilis Study has major influence on the willingness of minorities to participate in biomedical research. More individuals tended to hold a vague impression of having heard of a negative research study that would affect their trust in research and the government rather than a specific named event. The data from this study did show that 20% of blacks who said they did recall such an incident were able to describe the specifics or name the actual study. This was twice as common among blacks than among whites. Thus, these findings support the continuing importance of the Tuskegee Syphilis Study within the black community.

Institutional Review Boards

An IRB (institutional review board) is a federally mandated body established under the Department of Health and Human Services regulations for the protection of human subjects; information can be found at http://www.hhs.gov/ohrp/humansubjects/guidance/45cfr46.htm. Its purpose is to protect the rights and welfare of human subjects recruited to participate in research activities. The guiding ethical principles of the IRB are embodied in the Belmont Report discussed earlier in this chapter. The principles of respect for persons, beneficence, and justice are accepted as critical considerations for the ethical conduct of human subject research.

All research involving human subjects must be reviewed and approved by an organization's IRB prior to initiation of the research. This requirement applies to all human subject research conducted regardless of the funding support, if any, for the project.

Research involving human subjects includes the collection of data about or from human subjects (including surveys) and the use of existing data (including specimens). Any changes to a project after IRB approval must be submitted for review and approval before implementation. Continuing review is also required at regular intervals for certain protocols.

The IRB requires principal investigators and all other research team members to complete and document appropriate training in the protection of human subjects. Additionally, the IRB is tasked with monitoring ongoing research for adherence to federal regulations and institutional policies and procedures.

Each IRB has to have at least five members with varying backgrounds to promote complete and adequate review of research activities commonly conducted by the institution. The IRB must be sufficiently qualified through the experience and expertise of its members to ensure protection of human subjects in research activities. If an IRB regularly reviews research that involves a vulnerable category of subjects, such as children, prisoners, pregnant women, or handicapped or mentally disabled persons, consideration must be given to the inclusion of one or more individuals who are knowledgeable about and experienced in working with these subjects.

There are three levels of review: exempt from review, expedited review, and complete review. The IRB chairperson typically determines which level of review is required for each study.

Exempt Review

Studies that fall under any exempt category as defined by 45 CFR 46.101(b), may qualify for an exempt review. Principal investigator(s) whose research studies fall into one of the exemption categories typically submit an Application for Exempt Research to the Office of Compliance for review by the IRB. Along with the application, researchers should include a copy of the questionnaire, interview questions, survey outline, the cover/information letter, written description of any verbal instructions, and any other documentation that will be used.

Research that qualifies for exempt status does not require a signed informed consent form. It does require a written cover letter or information letter that informs the participants (human subjects) of what is expected of them. The cover letter or information letter should include the elements of informed consent.

The determination of an exempt status can be made by the IRB chairperson or designee identified by the IRB chairperson. Exemption cannot be granted for research that uses prisoners and for research with children that involves survey or interview procedures or observation of public behavior, unless the research involves observations of public behavior when the investigator(s) does not participate in the activities being observed. If the IRB finds the study is not exempt, it must go through an expedited or full board review. There are six categories that fall under the exempt status; they are summarized in **Table 8-4**. While research activities in which the only involvement of human subjects will be in one or more of Table 8-4's categories are exempt from the 45 CFR 46 regulations, they must still be submitted to the IRB for their review and approval.

Expedited Review

Research activities involving no more than minimal risk, and in which the only involvement of human subjects will be in one or more of the categories identified by 45 CFR 46.110, may be reviewed by the IRB through the expedited review procedure. **Table 8-5** lists the categories for expedited review. The expedited review procedure may not be used where identification of the subjects and/or their responses would reasonably place them at risk of criminal or civil liability. There must be evidence that reasonable and appropriate protections will be implemented so that risks related to invasion of privacy and breaches of confidentiality are no greater than minimal. An expedited review must be

Table 8-4   Categories of Exempt Research Activities

1. Educational Practices
   Research conducted in established or commonly accepted educational settings, involving normal educational practices, such as:
   a. research on regular and special educational instructional strategies, or
   b. research on the effectiveness of or the comparison among instructional techniques, curricula, or classroom management methods.

2. Surveys, Questionnaires, Interviews, Observational Studies
   Research involving the use of educational tests (cognitive, diagnostic, aptitude, achievement), survey procedures, interview procedures, or observation of public behavior unless:
   a. information obtained is recorded in such a manner that human subjects can be identified, directly or through identifiers linked to the subjects; and
   b. any disclosure of the human subjects' responses outside the research could reasonably place the subjects at risk of criminal or civil liability or be damaging to the subjects' financial standing, employability, or reputation.

3. Educational Tests
   Research involving the use of educational tests (cognitive, diagnostic, aptitude, achievement), survey procedures, interview procedures, or observation of public behavior, if:
   a. the human subjects are elected or appointed public officials or candidates for public office; or
   b. federal statue(s) require(s) without exception that the confidentiality of the personally identifiable information will be maintained throughout the research and thereafter.

4. Existing Data or Specimens
   Research involving the collection or study of existing data documents, records, pathological specimens, or diagnostic specimens, if these sources are publicly available or if the information is recorded by the investigator in such a manner that subjects cannot be identified, directly or through identifiers linked to the subjects.

5. Research and Demonstration Projects
   Research and demonstration projects which are conducted by or subject to the approval of department or agency heads, and which are designed to study, evaluate or otherwise examine:
   a. public benefit or service programs;
   b. procedures for obtaining benefits or services under those programs;
   c. possible changes in or alternatives to those programs or procedures; or
   d. possible changes in methods or levels of payment for benefits or services under those programs.

(continued)

Table 8-4   Categories of Exempt Research Activities *(continued)*

---

6. Taste and Food Quality and Consumer Acceptance
    Taste and food quality evaluation and consumer acceptance studies,
       a. if wholesome foods without additives are consumed, or
       b. if a food is consumed that contains a food ingredient at or below the level
          and for a use found to be safe, or agricultural chemical or environmental
          contaminant at or below the level found to be safe, by the Food and Drug
          Administration or approved by the Environmental Protection Agency
          or the Food Safety and Inspection Service of the U.S. Department of
          Agriculture.

Excerpted from http://research.nmsu.edu/compliance/IRB/forms.html

---

conducted by the IRB chairperson or by one or more of the experienced IRB members designated by the IRB chairperson from among members of the IRB in accordance with the requirements set forth in 45 CFR 46.110.

Full Board Review

Research that does not qualify for either exempt or expedited review must be reviewed by the full IRB. The full IRB review is conducted for studies that pose greater than minimal risk to human subjects. Investigators should ensure that risks are minimized and are reasonable in relation to anticipated benefits; they must also ensure equitable subject selection, documentation of informed consent, an adequate plan for monitoring data collection, and adequate provisions to protect privacy of participants and maintain confidentiality/anonymity of the data.

Are Ethical Violations a Thing of the Past?

You may be surprised to find out that the answer to this question is "no." In 2001, Ellen Roche died 1 month after receiving an experimental treatment of 1 g of hexamethonium to induce asthma-like effects. The pulmonary toxicity associated with hexamethonium had been published in several earlier reports that this investigation failed to locate (Perkins, 2001). Nicole Wan died after volunteering for a study on the effects of environmental air quality. The study involved undergoing a bronchoscopy to examine and collect lung cells. Because of continued discomfort during the procedure, Nicole received four times the maximum level of lidocaine. She suffered a cardiac arrest 3 hours

---

Table 8-5   Categories of Expedited Review

---

1. Clinical studies of drugs and medical devices only when condition (a) or (b) is met.
   a. Research on drugs for which an investigational new drug application (21 CFR Part 312) is not required. (Note: Research on marketed drugs that significantly increases the risks or decreases the acceptability of the risks associated with the use of the product is not eligible for expedited review.)
   b. Research on medical devices for which (1) an investigational device exemption application (21 CFR Part 812) is not required; or (2) the medical device is cleared/approved for marketing and the medical device is being used in accordance with its cleared/approved labeling.

2. Collection of blood samples by finger stick, heel stick, ear stick, or venipuncture as follows:
   a. From healthy, nonpregnant adults who weigh at least 110 pounds. For these subjects, the amounts drawn may not exceed 550 ml in an 8 week period and collection may not occur more frequently than 2 times per week; or
   b. From other adults and children*, considering the age, weight, and health of the subjects, the collection procedure, the amount of blood to be collected, and the frequency with which it will be collected. For these subjects, the amount drawn may not exceed the lesser of 50 ml or 3 ml per kg in an 8-week period and collection may not occur more frequently than 2 times per week.

3. Prospective collection of biological specimens for research purposes by noninvasive means. Examples include:
   a. hair and nail clippings in a nondisfiguring manner;
   b. deciduous teeth at time of exfoliation or if routine patient care indicates a need for extraction;
   c. permanent teeth if routine patient care indicates a need for extraction;
   d. excreta and external secretions (including sweat);
   e. uncannulated saliva collected either in an unstimulated fashion or stimulated by chewing gumbase or wax or by applying a dilute citric solution to the tongue;
   f. placenta removed at delivery;
   g. amniotic fluid obtained at the time of rupture of the membrance prior to or during labor;
   h. supra- and subgingival dental plaque and calculus, provided the collection procedure is not more invasive than routine prophylactic scaling of the teeth and the process is accomplished in accordance with accepted prophylactic techniques;
   i. mucosal and skin cells collected by buccal scraping or swab, skin swab, or mouth washings; and
   j. sputum collected after saline mist nebulization.

---

*Children are defined in the HHS regulations as "persons who have not attained the legal age for consent to treatments or procedures involved in the research, under the applicable law of the jurisdiction in which the research will be conducted." (45 CFR 46.402(a)). In New Mexico, the legal age for consent to treatments or procedures involved in the research is 18 years of age.

Table 8-5   Categories of Expedited Review *(continued)*

4. Collection of data through noninvasive procedures (not involving general anesthesia or sedation) routinely employed in clinical practice, excluding procedures involving x-rays or microwaves. Where medical devices are employed, they must be cleared/approved for marketing. (Studies intended to evaluate the safety and effectiveness of the medical device are not generally eligible for expedited review, including studies of cleared medical devices for new indications.) Examples include:
   a. physical sensors that are applied either to the surface of the body or at a distance and do not involve input of significant amounts of energy into the subject or an invasion of the subject's privacy;
   b. weighing or testing sensory acuity;
   c. magnetic resonance imaging;
   d. electrocardiography, electroencephalography, thermography, detection of naturally occurring radioactivity, electroretinography, ultrasound, diagnostic infrared imaging, doppler blood flow, and echocardiography; and
   e. moderate exercise, muscular strength testing, body composition assessment, and flexibility testing where appropriate given the age, weight, and health of the individual.

5. Research involving materials (data, documents, records, or specimens) that have been collected, or will be collected solely for nonresearch purposes (such as medical treatment or diagnosis). (Note: Some research in this category may be exempt from the HHS regulations for the protection of human subjects (45 CFR 46.101(b) (4)). This listing refers only to research that is not exempt.

6. Collection of data from voice, video, digital, or image recordings made for research purposes.

7. Research on individual or group characteristics or behavior (including, but not limited to, research on perception, cognition, motivation, identity, language, communication, cultural beliefs or practices, and social behavior) or research employing survey interview, oral history, focus group, program evaluation, human factors evaluation, or quality assurance methodologies. (Note: Some research in this category may be exempt from the HHS regulations for the protection of human subjects (45 CFR 46.101(b) (2) and (b) (3)). This listing refers only to research that is not exempt.

8. Continuing review of research previously approved by the convened IRB as follows:
   a. where (1) the research is permanently closed to the enrollment of new subjects; (2) all subjects have completed all research-related interventions; and (3) the research remains active only for long-term follow-up of subjects; or
   b. where no subjects have been enrolled and no additional risks have been identified; or
   c. where the remaining research activities are limited to data analysis.

9. Continuing review of research, not conducted under an investigational new drug application or investigational device exemption where categories two (2) through eight (8) do not apply but the IRB has determined and documented at a convened meeting that the research involves no greater than minimal risk and no additional risks have been identified.

Excerpted from http://research.nmsu.edu/compliance/IRB/forms.html

later and died 2 days later (retrieved February 28, 2010 from http://tech.mit.edu/V116/N17/rochester.17n.html). Ethical considerations in respondent sampling (also called snowball sampling) in HIV/AIDS biobehavioral surveys in Lebanon are discussed in DeJong et al. (2009). Ethical issues such as monetary incentives, social stigma associated with participating, and confidentiality breeches are discussed.

A further example of ethical violations involving an organization's IRB is provided by the Johns Hopkins University/Kennedy Krieger Institute (KKI) lead paint study. Bozeman, Slade, and Hirsch (2009) compare what went wrong during the Tuskegee Syphilis Study with violations made during the KKI lead paint study. The authors discuss lessons learned or not learned since the Tuskegee Syphilis Study. During the 1992 KKI lead paint study, minority children were purposely exposed to lead to study its effects. Further, researchers encouraged proprietors of the homes known to have lead paint to rent to families with young children. In 1992, the negative effects of lead on children (mental retardation and other brain disorders) were widely known. However, this study was approved by the two institutions' IRBs. How could this have happened given all of the laws, institutional guidelines, and formal professional ethics developed since the Tuskegee study? Ethical violations of the study point to an overdependence on institutionalized science ethics as a prevention for such catastrophes. While not advocating for the absence of review boards, the authors do advocate for more transparent IRB review and a process to identify problem areas. They believe more could have been learned from this ethical disgrace by an analysis of the deliberations of the IRB during review of this research proposal. They state that "clearly something in the composition, formation, management, or deliberation of the IRBs is problematic to say the least and potentially disastrous at its worst" (Bozeman et al., 2009).

ETHICS IN EVIDENCE-BASED NURSING PRACTICE

Relationship Between Ethics in Nursing Research and Ethics in Evidence-Based Nursing Practice

If we revisit Chaloner's (2007) definition of ethics once more, we see that "ethics is a branch of philosophy concerned with determining right and wrong in relation to people's decisions and actions." This can also apply to evidence-based nursing practice (EBNP). Evidence-based nursing practice reflects a paradigm shift in how nursing practice is taught, practiced and evaluated (Milton, 2007). She shares that it is no longer acceptable for nurses to continue doing things the way they have always been done without being able to back up their actions based on best available evidence. Areas of current debate include the process of selecting evidence, what should be included as evidence, how much emphasis should any one type of evidence receive in the overall evidence synthesis, and the potential lack of holistic but individualized patient care. Incorporating patient values and available clinical expertise can be quite subjective in nature and dependent on the nurse participating in EBNP.

Potential Ethical Pitfalls in Evidence-Based Nursing Practice

Narrow Scope of What Constitutes "Evidence"

Evidence-based practice (EBP) definitions are varied but all include evidence from three broad areas: empirical studies, other forms of published evidence (e.g., review articles, clinical pathways, and protocols), available clinical expertise and resources, and patient preferences/nuisances. Historically, evidence from randomized controlled trials (RCTs) and systematic reviews have taken the honor of being on top of the evidence hierarchy (Pearson, Wiechula, Court, & Lockwood, 2007; Milton, 2007; Rycroft-Malone et al., 2004; Bolton, 2001). Archie Cochrane is noted for founding the Cochrane Collaboration, an international, nonprofit organization that focuses on collecting and updating evidence. The Cochrane Collaboration considers the RCT as the gold standard of research evidence (Milton, 2007). However, the ability of the RCT to predict cause and effect relationships and reduce potential biases from extraneous variables has limited its ability to mimic the real world and real life situations.

Given the limitations of the RCT and the most current literature, it makes sense to suggest using a broader evidence base, which includes not only empirical quantitative studies but also qualitative research studies, clinical experience, patient experience, and information from the local context/organizational culture (Rycroft-Malone et al., 2004). Qualitative research is increasingly recognized as a credible form of evidence in evidence-based nursing practice. Qualitative nursing research contributes to EBNP by adding the subjective, intuitive evidence that is so much a part of nursing practice. As Milton (2007) shares, "Health is never objective, classified, or judged. Instead, it is described by the person who is living in it, and can only be described by the person living it. Thus, the goal of nursing is health and quality of life from the healthcare recipient's perspective."

Even though nurses draw on a diversity of information sources to provide care to their patients, patients' experiences/preferences and clinical experience have largely been ignored. Knowledge from clinical experience is often tacit and intuitive and has been hard to articulate. The gathering and interpretation of individuals' values, experiences, and preferences into evidence-based practice is a skill that is complex but can be learned. One of the most difficult challenges is when the scientific evidence (in both qualitative and quantitative studies) does not fit well with the human evidence (clinical experience and patient values). Rycroft-Malone et al. (2004) shares the example of the recommendation to use compression bandaging to treat venous leg ulcers. However, the individual patient may refuse this "best practice treatment" because of the discomfort caused by the bandaging. A second example is provided by Griffitt (2008), who shared a personal clinical experience involving a hospitalized elderly woman with dementia from an area nursing home. Aggressive, sometimes painful but competent nursing care had been provided over several weeks in several settings, but no one had stepped back to look at the bigger picture to identify the patient's goals and values. Griffitt was able to talk to the daughter and find out that this aggressive treatment was not respectful of her mother's choices.

Integrating all types of empirical research (scientific approach) with clinical experience and patient values (intuitive approach) is challenging but worth the result of quality patient care. Pearson et al. (2007) also support this idea by advocating for the inclusion of diverse forms of evidence including all forms of empirical research, expert opinion, and clinical experience. Pearson et al. also discuss how the Joanna Briggs Institute (JBI) model of evidence-based health care conceptualizes evidence-based practice in this way. They also support the assumption that no particular form of evidence has overall superiority. Whatever the form of evidence, the critical point is that it should be subjected to scrutiny through critique and analysis (Rycroft-Malone et al., 2004). The JBI model of evidence-based health care identifies four major evidence interests of clinicians: evidence of feasibility, evidence of appropriateness, evidence of meaningfulness, and evidence of effectiveness. Feasibility issues such as costs, adequate resources, organizational culture that is supportive, and practicality must be considered when involved in evidence-based health care. Appropriateness refers to how the intervention fits with the situation both culturally and ethically. Meaningfulness relates to how relevant the intervention is to the patient, and effectiveness is to what degree the intervention produced the desired effect. Using these four major evidence interests to integrate and synthesize across all forms of evidence allows the emphasis to be placed accordingly. This results in a dynamic process that can change depending on the circumstances of these four areas of interest. The 10 steps of evidence-based nursing practice developed by this author incorporate all forms of acceptable evidence and these evidence interests as identified by the JBI model of evidence-based health care.

A Cookbook Approach

By choosing to focus exclusively on randomized controlled trials (RCT), nursing practice becomes reduced to standard step-by-step cookbook instructions for patient care. While possibly reducing costs and improving healthcare services, this approach may serve more to harm the individual patient rather than help them (Milton, 2007).

To prevent evidence-based nursing practice from being "cookbook" nursing, the nurse must decide how to incorporate patient preferences/values into the practice change for any particular patient (DiCenso, Cullum, & Ciliska, 1998). These authors suggest that the incorporation of clinical expertise be balanced with the risks and benefits of treatment options for each patient. Further, there is a need to take into account the patient's unique circumstances such as co-morbid conditions and preferences (DiCenso, Cullum, & Ciliska, 1998).

Policy makers, health managers, and health insurance companies may have the expectation that once sound evidence about the best treatment for a particular health problem is identified, all providers should treat all patients in the same way, eliminating variability in treatment and costs (Shorten & Wallace, 1997). This is a very limited and risky way to approach evidence-based practice. Further, if patients' values and needs are not considered along with the scientific evidence from the beginning, issues of noncompliance, mistrust, and alienation of the patient may very well occur. To be evidence-based nursing practice, variability in treatment is an expected outcome. Lack of variability would support the cookbook approach of one size fits all and positive outcomes would be questionable.

A clinical scenario shared by one of my nursing students provides a practical, simple illustration of how evidence-based practice can incorporate personal values and needs into care.

> The nurses on my unit start and discontinue IVs throughout the day. Hand gel dispensers are in every IV tray, on the walls behind each patient bed, and located at the nurses' station. It is policy to use the hand gel before and after patient contact *within the patient's eyesight*. This ensures that our patients know we are clean and serious about their care.
>
> A few weeks ago one of my patients was watching me race back and forth between the other patients. He commented that I must go through a couple bottles of hand gel every day. He then asked me how the hand gel works. I explained that the hand gel was alcohol based and using it while rubbing one's hands together kills the germs on one's hands. He replied that he thought hand gel was a sham. I provided the patient with information about hand gel, hoping this would relieve his doubts. It did not. Before I took out his IV, I thoroughly washed my hands using soap and water. He laughed and thanked me for doing so.
>
> I know that evidence-based nursing practice shows hand gel is sufficient during patient care until the hands start to feel thick or sticky (usually around the fifth application). I also realized that the patient was uncomfortable, and although I attempted to educate him, I eventually changed my practice to give individualized care, thereby satisfying him (B. Lee, personal communication, March 2, 2010).

Cost Versus Quality

It has been argued that evidence-based practice has emerged in response to the rising cost of health care. Some references even go as far as to indicate that its sole purpose was to ration treatment and/or reduce costs (Smith, 1998; Shorten & Wallace, 1997). Milton (2007) states that EBP arose from an economic need to determine the cost/benefit ratio of treatments as a way to contain healthcare costs. Good quality evidence may support not only effective interventions but also cost-effective ones. However, cost is just one factor to consider and should not be the driving force behind evidence-based practice.

REFERENCES

Bolton, J. (2001). The evidence in evidence-based practice: What counts and what doesn't count? *Journal of Manipulative and Physiological Therapeutics, 24*, 362–366.

Bozeman, B., Slade, C., & Hirsch, P. (2009). Understanding bureaucracy in health science ethics: Toward a better institutional review board. *American Journal of Public Health, 99*, 1549–1556.

Chaloner, C. (2007). An introduction to ethics in nursing, *Nursing Standard, 21*, 42–45.

DeJong, J. (2009). Ethical considerations in HIV/AIDS biobehavioral surveys that use respondent-driven sampling: Illustrations from Lebanon. *American Journal of Public Health, 99*, 1562–1567.

DiCenso, A., Cullum, N., & Ciliska, D. (1998). Implementing evidence-based nursing: Some misconceptions. *Evidence-Based Nursing, 1*, 38–39.

Griffitt, R. (2008). Letters to the editor. *Nursing Science Quarterly, 21*, 183–184.

IRB Guidebook. (n.d.). Retrieved from http://www.hhs.gov/ohrp/irb/irb_appendices.htm#j7.

Jones, J. (1993). *Bad blood: The Tuskegee Syphilis Study.* New York, NY: The Free Press.

Katz, R., Jean-Charles, G., Green, B., Kressin, N., Claudio, C., Wang, M., et al. (2009). Identifying the Tuskegee Syphilis Study: Implications of results from recall and recognition questions. *BMC Public Health, 9*, 468.

McGuire, D. (1996, April 9). Rochester death halts MIT-funded study. *The TECH Online Edition (Cambridge, Massachusetts), 116*(17). Retrieved from http://tech.mit.edu/V116/N17/rochester.17n.html.

Milton, C. (2007). Evidence-based practice: Ethical questions for nursing. *Nursing Science Quarterly, 20*, 123–126.

Nieswiadomy, R. (2008). *Foundations of nursing research* (5th ed.). Upper Saddle River, NJ: Pearson-Prentice Hall.

Pearson, A., Wiechula, R., Court, A., & Lockwood, C. (2007). A reconsideration of what constitutes "evidence" in the healthcare professions. *Nursing Science Quarterly, 20*, 85–88.

Perkins, E. (2001). Johns Hopkins' tragedy: Could librarians have prevented a death? *NewsBreaks and The Weekly News Digest.* Retrieved from http://newsbreaks.infotoday.com/nbreader.asp?ArticleID=17534.

Reverby, S. (2000). Introduction: More than a metaphor. *Tuskegee Truths: Rethinking The Tuskegee Syphilis Study* (pp. 1–14). Chapel Hill, NC: University of North Carolina Press.

Rycroft-Malone, J., Seers, K., Titchen, A., Harvey, G., Kitson, A., & McCormack, B. (2004). What counts as evidence in evidence-based practice? *Nursing and Health Care Management and Policy, 47,* 81–90.

Shorten, A., & Wallace, M. (1997). Evidence-based practice: When quality counts. *Australian Nursing Journal, 4,* 26–27.

Silva, M. (1995). *Ethical guidelines in the conduct, dissemination, and implementation of nursing research.* Washington, DC: American Nurses Association.

Smith, J. (1998). Conference report: exploring evidence based practice: International conference organized by the University of Southhampton School of Nursing and Midwifery at the Chilworth Manor Conference Centre, Southhampton England, 12–14 September 1997. *Journal of Advanced Nursing, 27,* 227–229.

Strait, G. (1993). *The deadly deception.* Television program produced by NOVA and PBS.

USDHHS (2003). *Health information privacy.* Retrieved from http://www.hhs.gov/ocr/privacy/hipaa/understanding/special/research/index.html.

World Medical Association Declaration of Helsinki: Ethical Principles for Medical Research Involving Human Subjects. Retrieved from http://ohsr.od.nih.gov/guidelines/helsinki.html.

CHAPTER 9

Evidence-Based Nursing Practice Projects: Putting It All Together

TIME TO GET DOING

Congratulations! You now have all of the tools you need to participate in evidence-based nursing practice! I have discussed important concepts such as nursing research, the research process, research utilization, and evidence-based nursing practice (EBNP). In Chapter 5, steps were presented for creating EBNP changes to improve the quality of your patient's care. The topic of Chapter 6 was how to analyze empirical research studies. Critique examples were included. All of the aforementioned information is important for this next step of creating and implementing evidence-based nursing practice. Two detailed examples of EBNP projects are presented here to take you through each step of the EBNP process. The first problem examined is dissatisfaction with visitation policy in critical care by family members (Gary, 2007). The second problem is surgical site infection (Lyons, Hamburg, Holden, Arumugam, & Book, 2009).

Identifying the Practice Problem/Issue

In the first problem identified by Gary (2007), dissatisfaction with the current visitation policy in critical care by family members was the focus. If we take the questions provided in Chapter 5 to clarify and refine the problem, we have the following information:

- Do I want to focus on prevention or treatment? **Treatment of the current dissatisfaction by family members**
- What population am I focusing on? (e.g., elderly, cognitively impaired, physically handicapped) **Critically ill patients**
- What setting am I interested in? (e.g., hospital, long-term care facility, home) **Critical care settings in hospitals**

- What is the current problem? **Families and patients are verbally complaining about the current visitation policy as being too restricted. Family members state that the current policy does not allow flexibility to adapt to conflicting work and life schedules.**
- What is the current policy and is it being followed? **Current policy allows only immediate family to visit four times a day (two 30-minute and two 1-hour visitation sessions) and is limited to only four visitors at the bedside at a time. Nurses are currently following the policy.**
- How will I individualize the intervention or practice change? **Establishment of individual visiting preferences with patient's input and identification of a special care partner allowed at all hours if desired by the patient**

Therefore, the problem statement becomes, **"Restrictive visitation policy for critical care families related to current policy only allows immediate family to visit four times a day as evidenced by family and patients complaints."**

Collecting and Appraising the Evidence

Empirical Evidence

Empirical evidence is actual research studies that may include a combination of clinical trials, nonexperimental level research, and systematic reviews/meta-analyses. Descriptions are found in Chapter 5. To support a solution for the problem of restricted critical care visitation, Gary (2007) shares three primary research studies.

Roland, Russell, Richards, & Sullivan (2001) show that a less restrictive visitation policy developed and implemented with nursing input proved satisfactory for patients, family, and healthcare staff. Findings resulted in positive improvements such as increased family and patient perceptions of quality of care, decrease in complaints, increased family involvement with care, and increased communication between family and staff. The authors recommended that nurses be involved in the decision-making process of visitation policy to incorporate their ideas and to obtain buy-in from potentially resistant staff. Livesay et al. (2005) examined visitation policy after nurses questioned the effects of open visitation on neuroscience patients. Nurses were surveyed about their attitudes toward visitation in a neurosurgery ICU. Based on the variability in nurses' interpretation and implementation of individualized open visitation policies, suggestions included staff education about the policy and its implementation, a review of the literature to determine the validity of concerns about deleterious physiologic effects on neuroscience patients from visitation, and improved communication among nurses about visitation.

Lee et al. (2007) support the role played by families in a critically ill patient's recovery. In a two-part study, the authors surveyed the visiting policies of New England-area ICUs and used nursing focus groups to describe the challenges and barriers that nursing staff working in open visitation ICU settings experience in order to provide solutions for assisting in the implementation of such policies for other facilities. Results indicated that restricted visiting hours in the intensive care unit increase anxiety and dissatisfaction in both critically ill patients and their families.

Nonempirical Evidence

Nonempirical evidence includes published reviews and protocols/guidelines. An example of a review article that Gary (2007) included was a review by Sims & Miracle (2006). Review of research over the perceived barriers and benefits to open visitation was presented. Perceived barriers by nurses included the belief that visitation is too tiring for the patient and could be physiologically harmful to the patient by increasing heart rate and blood pressure; that it impedes delivery of nursing and medical care; and/or that family members become tired if they visit too much. However, research has demonstrated that there are many benefits to flexible visitation for patients, families, and staff. Benefits include reduction of anxiety in the patient; flexibility of when the family can visit accommodating their busy lifestyles; better communication between the family and staff; support for the patient; decrease in cardiovascular complications by decreasing heart rate, blood pressure, and intracranial pressure; and actual promotion of the patient's rest. White and Edwards (2006) published example visitation guidelines. These guidelines were developed from a research-based family-centered approach to visitation. Input from patients, caregivers, security, and administration using a team approach was used to develop these guidelines. Highlights from the visitation guidelines included such things as visiting hours from 9 a.m. to 9 p.m. with no more than two visitors in the room at a time. Visits were not to exceed 30 minutes unless the patient desired a longer visit. Another example was the establishment of individual visiting preferences with patient's input and identification of a special care partner allowed at all hours if desired by the patient.

In fact, Berwick and Kotagal (2004) state that restricting visiting in critical care is not caring, compassionate, or necessary. Further, they advised that a more liberal policy may help by providing a support system and a familiar environment as well as by creating trust between families and care providers. The

AACN also supports replacing strict, inflexible visitation policies with policies that offer a more flexible, individualized approach (Sims & Miracle, 2006).

Reading and Critically Analyzing Empirical Research for Evidence

It is important not to forget that the empirical evidence must be analyzed for strengths and limitations using the criteria provided in Chapter 4. To be included as relevant evidence, the study should score an overall ranking of Fair or better.

Summarizing Across the Evidence

At this point, it is necessary to summarize across all available evidence obtained, including empirical and nonempirical evidence. Synthesize the findings from the evidence you have deemed credible. As discussed in Chapter 5, this is done very similarly to what is called content analysis. Used in this context, content analysis involves examining the findings for recurrent themes across the studies or the majority of studies. As discussed earlier, it is very dangerous to base a practice change on a single study. However, if you find that multiple studies are proposing the same practice change, then you can start to feel more confident in proposing this change. If themes are not evident, then you need to decide carefully whether to continue with the EBNP process or stop at this point and consider further investigation and research first. It might be that there is not enough evidence to support a practice change. Rather, the evidence or lack thereof is supporting the need for more research first.

In the current example, the most significant theme was the need for a more liberal visitation policy in the critical care areas. However, what was not clear was how that liberal visitation policy was to be operationalized at the unit level. White and Edwards (2006) offered the most detailed suggestions in their article on visitation guidelines discussed previously. Thus, current evidence supports a less restrictive visitation policy and provides some idea of what that policy could look like. However, evidence also supports the need to include all parties impacted from such a practice change—including family members and patients—in the policy development.

Integrating the Evidence with Clinical Expertise and Client Preferences and Values

The next level of evidence to be synthesized and added is clinical expertise and patient preferences and values. Clinical expertise is obtained through expert interviews and current best practice guidelines. To incorporate patient needs and preferences, individual or group interviews can be conducted with past critical care patients and their families. Another method would be a mailed-out survey to patients and their families asking their opinions. Experts can be identified by their clinical expertise in the topic/problem area of focus. To ensure a thorough analysis of clinical expertise available, a multidisciplinary approach should be used. For the issue of dissatisfaction with the current hospital policy on visitation in the critical care units, experts might include representation from staff nurses who work in this area, someone from administration, someone from security and/or patient safety, a recent family member and/or patient, hospital chaplain, and physician. In this particular case, a meeting could be held to ask everyone for his or her input and expert opinion regarding the issue. To facilitate synthesis and identification of themes across expert interviews, you need to develop a slate of questions to use for all interviews. Sample interview questions were presented in Table 5-2 and are presented again here in **Table 9-1**. As you can see, these questions are general and could be easily adapted to each specific issue. For example, with the current issue of visitation policy in the critical care area, one of the questions that can be asked is, "What has been your experience with the current critical care visitation policy?" In addition, "What do you think the current best practice is for visitation in critical care areas?"

Developing the Proposed Practice Change in Detail

Once all of the evidence is critically analyzed and synthesized, you should have some good ideas for what to propose as an intervention or practice change. Representation by the target population in the development of the practice change is critical for buy-in and success of the change. These individuals can serve as champions for implementation and ultimate success of your project. This step is the point where decisions are made about who will receive the practice change, what it will entail, when it will happen, where it will take place, and how it will take place.

In the current example, the "who" would be everyone impacted by a new critical care visitation policy. This may include critical care staff nurses, physicians, administration, patients, family members, clergy, safety officers, to name just a few people that may be affected by such as practice change. The "what" would be the development of an effective visitation policy that all could agree upon and support. Ideally, representation from these areas would have served on a committee early on in the practice change inception. Evidence collection, analysis, and synthesis might have been started by one nurse but for an organizational change to occur would need to have been extended to all parties with a vested interest (stakeholders) to achieve buy-in. Once the key ingredients to a policy change were agreed to, implementation and evaluation of the new policy could be done.

To obtain buy-in from the rest of involved staff, an educational session could be offered. However, this should not be the first communication with

Table 9-1   Sample Interview Questions to Assess Patient Preferences and Clinical Expertise

Sample Questions for Patients/Clients

How long have you been dealing with this problem? (You can go ahead and state specifically what the problem is.)

What things have you tried to help deal with the _____ (problem)? How well have they worked?

What suggestions/treatments have been used by your healthcare provider to help with this problem?

Can you give any examples of what has worked and what has not worked for you personally?

Sample Questions for Experts

Find out credentials, years of experience, and where these years have been spent.

Do not use actual names of experts; use initials or fake names.

What has been your experience with _____ (condition/problem)?

Do you have any successful case studies/scenarios that you can share related to this experience?

What do you think the current best practice is for dealing with this _____ (condition/problem)?

What do you base this answer on? (e.g., research, policies, protocols, providers, etc.)

Is this current best practice you speak of being used in your facility/organization?

If not, why do you think it is not being used? If so, how is it going? How is it being evaluated/how are outcomes measured?

Would you say that your organization currently uses evidence-based practice? If not, why not? If so, can you give an example especially with _____ (condition/problem)?

those impacted by such a practice change. Initial communication and requesting ideas to solve the problem/issue could be done by focus groups or written survey. Newsletters, emails, and bulletin boards are methods that could be used to keep staff informed throughout the process along with encouraging ideas and feedback that could be taken back to the visitation policy committee for review and consideration.

An outline of the educational content would then be developed based on research findings. Timing of delivery of the education would be the next step to plan. For example, will it be a mandatory educational session for all staff in the critical care units or just the nurses? Will they get paid to attend? How many times will it need to be offered so that target audience can attend? How will compliance to attending be monitored? Next, are decisions about "where" it will take place. Is there a large enough room close to the target audience? Are there costs involved in using the location? Decisions about who will conduct the sessions, length of sessions, provision of refreshments or door prizes, and advertisement and marketing decisions will need to be made.

The "how" of the practice change implementation would include the process leading up to and throughout the actual implementation of the education. Timing of implementation of any new practice change is critical for its success. Nursing administration and nursing staff within the critical care areas would need to be queried as to when implementation might be the most successful. Selected staff should be identified to become champions for successful implementation of the new practice change. Formal and informal leaders from the staff should be carefully selected to move the impetus toward successful change.

Feasibility Issues

Feasibility issues include costs, time, and needed resources. A budget, timeline, and list of needed resources should be identified. For the current issue of implementation of new visitation policy, the following costs would need to be calculated:

Development of the visitation policy committee:

- Communication costs (mail, phone calls, flyers, posters)
- Salary for any committee members that are staff to attend meetings
- Refreshments for meetings
- Room to have meetings
- Resources to retrieve the needed evidence (librarian, computer data bases, copying costs)

Implementation of the visitation policy:

- Salaries for staff to attend educational sessions
- Costs of marketing the policy change
- Room to have educational sessions
- Refreshments if any during educational sessions
- Pre- and posttest survey regarding knowledge and attitudes over the issue

Evaluation of the visitation policy:

- Nurse and patient/family satisfaction surveys
- Cost, time, and room to conduct staff focus groups
- Salary of personnel tasked to collect, analyze, and report outcome data

Evaluating the Practice Change

Outcome measures must be identified in order to evaluate the effectiveness of any practice change. For this example, to determine initial knowledge and attitudes of staff, pre- and posttest surveys would be conducted at the educational session. Three months after implementation of the new policy, a written satisfaction survey would be conducted with both nurses and patients/families to see how well they liked the visitation policy. Further, focus groups with staff/nurses and a sample of individual patient/family interviews could be done. Based on the results of these outcomes, the visitation policy would continue as initially implemented or be revised if satisfaction had not improved. Six months later, outcomes would be measured again and action taken if needed. Then, collection of outcomes would occur on an annual basis.

Marketing the Practice Change

Marketing and obtaining buy-in for the practice change are crucial to its success. Including representation from all stakeholders from the inception of any practice change idea will facilitate adoption of the change. Communication is critical in marketing the visitation policy. Keeping stakeholders informed throughout the process, asking for feedback, encouraging positive talk among the rest of the staff that will be involved, getting administrative support, and publicizing the positives that the change will cause are all ideas to consider. The most effective mode of communication is word of mouth using champions for the cause. Other strategies include email, posters, flyers, notice of planning meetings, and encouragement of anyone concerned or interested to attend.

Strategies for Successful Implementation

Strategies for successful implementation include many of the aforementioned ideas. Key strategies include the right visitation policy committee, effective communication and marketing strategies, obtaining feedback from key stakeholders, comprehensive review and synthesis of available evidence, and saturation of dissemination of the practice change. Following the steps of the EBNP process as described here will facilitate adoption and integration of the practice change. Knowledge of the principles of planned change will help you anticipate barriers that may occur. Planned change in general is covered in Chapter 10. For this specific example, Gary (2007) used Lewin's Theory of Change. As Gary shares:

> In utilizing Lewin's theory for policy change in visitation, the stage of unfreezing requires motivation to promote change in practice. An awareness of the need for change is presented as well as the diagnosis of the problem with possible solutions created by the committee. This need for change is taken from surveys of

patient and family satisfaction with current critical care visitation polices and research. The committee can start formulating the framework for the change process and address specific forces that will facilitate change as well as impede change. According to Lewin, the committee must overcome the restraining forces by strengthening the driving forces in order for change to occur (Buonocore, 2004). Documenting this information in a proposal format will serve to solidify the thought process (Buonocore). In the stage of moving, the change is in process. For this visitation policy change, a trial period of 6 months will be used for implementation of the proposed change and evaluated by the same survey method mentioned prior. In the stage of refreezing, the new change is integrated into policy and over time the changes will become part of the hospital's values of delivering complete, person-centered, community-focused health care.

Sustainability of Practice Change

Continued monitoring and reinforcement of the practice change is important for sustainability. As mentioned, outcomes will be measured at 3 months, 6 months, and then at yearly intervals to determine the level of success of the new visitation policy in the critical care area. Educational sessions can be done on a yearly basis with staff and included in new employee orientation. A brochure can be developed to inform family and patients about the current visitation policy. Nurses can explain and answer any questions the patient or family may have on admission to the critical care unit regarding the policy. It is imperative that the change in practice stays current and continues to be supported by the evidence. At a minimum, a search for any new evidence needs to be completed on an annual basis. This evidence needs to be evaluated and synthesized and the current policy revised accordingly.

Okay, ready to develop another EBNP project? We will use the same approach and steps as we just did in the visitation policy earlier.

Identifying the Practice Problem/Issue

In this example, surgical site infection is the problem (Lyons, Hamburg, Bolden, Arumugam, & Book, 2009). If we take the questions provided in Chapter 5 to clarify and refine the problem, we have the following information:

- Do I want to focus on prevention or treatment? **Prevention of surgical site infection**
- What population am I focusing on? (e.g., elderly, cognitively impaired, physically handicapped) **Surgical patients**
- What setting am I interested in? (e.g., hospital, long-term care facility, home) **Hospitals and settings where surgeries are performed**
- What is the current problem? **According to Johns Hopkins Medicine's Center for Innovation in Quality Patient Care (2009), "Infections at surgical sites complicate about 780,000 procedures annually, or**

more than 1 in 40." According to Koopman et al. (2007), patients with surgical site infections are twice as likely to die, 60% more likely to be admitted to intensive care units, and have higher rates of hospital readmissions than those patients that do not develop one. Healthcare cost for patients with a surgical site infection are approximately $5,000 more per patient than those who do not develop a surgical site infection (Koopman et al., 2007).

- What is the current policy and is it being followed? **Current policy lacks comprehensiveness and does not address all recommended measures by the surgical care improvement project sponsored by The Joint Commission (The Joint Commission, 2009).**

- How will I individualize the intervention or practice change? **Tailored education to patients and families on prevention of surgical site infections; using appropriate prophylactic antibiotics based on surgical procedure, implementing individual means to maintain normothermia (warmed blankets, Bair Hugger blanket, and warm packs) and normoglycemia (insulin therapy as needed). Establishment of huddle rounds to include the individual patient and their family in the plan of care is critical to the success of preventing surgical site infections (Blum, 2009).**

Therefore, the problem statement becomes, **"Surgical site infections related to lack of implementation of evidence-based guidelines are evidenced by high rates of surgical site infections and increased morbidity and mortality associated with these high rates."**

Collecting and Appraising the Evidence

Empirical Evidence

To support a solution for the problem of surgical site infection, Lyons et al. (2007) share nine primary research studies (seven quantitative and two qualitative studies) that relate to the topic. Findings and recommendations to reduce surgical site infections from three of these studies follow.

Rhee and Harris (2008) focused on adequate skin antisepsis as a way to reduce surgical site infections. This was a 1-year observational pilot study initiated to evaluate the effects of a prepackaged 2% chlorhexidine gluconate (CHG) impregnated no-rinse cloth on the rate of surgical site infections. Participants received instructions both verbally and in writing from the preoperative nurse. The nurse provided assistance if needed. During the year prior to the study, 5174 procedures resulted in a surgical site infection rate of 2.1%. At the end of the study, 4266 procedures resulted in a surgical site infection rate of 0.7%. Cost savings from readmission were $177,937. Average cost due to surgical site infections was $648,471 preintervention and $290,827 postintervention. Thus, using this prepackaged 2% CHG cloth was highly effective in reducing the rate of surgical site infections, which resulted in significant cost savings and reduction in patient morbidity and mortality.

DeBaun (2008) also provides support for using a 2% CHG solution in reducing the rate of surgical site infections. Her study adds to Rhee and Harris (2008) discussed previously in that she found that an alcohol-free 2% CHG solution was effective against selected strains of multidrug resistant (MDR) and methicillin-resistant *Staphylococcus aureus* (MRSA) organisms.

Melling, Ali, Scott, and Leaper (2001) used a randomized controlled trial to examine the effects of preoperative warming on the incidence of wound infection after surgery. Patients (N = 421) having clean (breast, varicose vein, or hernia) surgery were randomly assigned to a nonwarmed group or one of two warmed groups (local and systemic). An intention to treat was used as a basis for the analysis. Significantly, lower wound infections were found in the warmed groups (5%) than in the nonwarmed patients (14%). No significant differences were found between the two warming groups (local versus systemic). This study supports that warming patients before clean surgery aids in the prevention of postoperative wound infection.

Nonempirical Evidence

Nonempirical evidence includes published reviews and protocols/guidelines. For surgical site infections, much progress has been made in the development of established standards and protocols. Major players in these initiatives include The Joint Commission (formerly JCAHO), Surgical Care Improvement Project (SCIP), and the Centers for Disease Control (CDC). Surgical site infection is identified as a National Patient Safety Goal that requires hospitals to "implement evidence-based practices for preventing surgical site infections" (JCAHO, 2009). Methods important to JCAHO in the reduction of surgical site infections include:

- Continuing education of healthcare providers
- Education of families and patients about surgical site infection and its prevention
- Creation of policies and protocols dedicated to the prevention of surgical site infection and adherence to the standards set forth by the CDC
- Conduction of periodic risk assessments, monitoring of compliance with evidence-based practice guidelines, and evaluation of the effectiveness of these guidelines
- Measuring surgical site infection rates for the first 30 days following procedures that do not involve inserting implantable devices and for the first year for those that do

The Surgical Care Improvement Project (SCIP) incorporates a partnership of organizations that are interested in improving surgical care by significantly reducing surgical complications (JCAHO, 2009). SCIP includes 10 healthcare agencies dedicated to eradicating surgical site infections. The healthcare agencies involved include:

- Agency for Healthcare Research and Quality
- American College of Surgeons
- American Hospital Association
- American Society of Anesthesiologists
- Association of Preoperative Registered Nurses
- Centers for Disease Control
- Institute for Healthcare Improvement
- The Joint Commission
- Veterans Health Administration
- Centers for Medicare and Medicaid Services

Recommendations by SCIP for preventing surgical site infections include:

- Prophylactic antibiotics at 1 hour preincision
- Tailored selection of antibiotic based on the procedure and individual needs of each patient
- Discontinuance of prophylactic antibiotic within 24 hours postincision; exception is the cardiac patient who should have these discontinued 48 hours postoperatively
- Appropriate hair removal (i.e., clipping)
- Normothermia

Other nonempirical sources substantiate the above recommendations or add to them. For example, Haycock et al. (2005) describes the recommended choice of antibiotics prior to cardiac surgery as cefazolin 1 g. Depending on the type of medication, the Centers for Disease Control recommend administration of prophylactic antibiotic medication one hour preincision to achieve the right concentration (Hobson, 2009). For most procedures, prophylactic antibiotics should be discontinued within 24 hours of the surgery end time. For cardiac surgeries, this time has been extended to 48 hours based on input and evidence supported by groups such as the Society of Thoracic Surgeons (Daniels, 2007). Hobson's review article (2009) discusses the negative effects of shaving with a razor, including small nicks created in the skin allowing organisms to colonize and lead to infection. Recommendations include not removing hair any sooner than 2 hours prior to surgery and preferably with use of electric clippers. Management of patient's blood sugar levels is related to a decrease in surgical site infections. An insulin protocol was tested with cardiac surgery patients that resulted in an aggressive approach in returning patients to

a normal blood sugar range. The average time to target range for this population was 5.2 hours (Haycock et al., 2005). Hsieh et al. (2006) recommend that
the length of time spent on surgical hand scrubs should last approximately 5
minutes and report that the CDC strongly recommends that when performing
surgical hand scrubs, providers should follow manufacturers' written directions for scrubbing duration, usually 2–6 minutes.

Reading and Critically Analyzing Empirical Research for Evidence

As mentioned before, it is important not to forget that the empirical evidence
must be analyzed for strengths and limitations using the criteria provided in
Chapter 6. To be included as relevant evidence, the study should score an overall ranking of Fair or better.

Summarizing Across the Evidence

Summarizing across the evidence is critical in identifying recurrent themes and
recommendations to solve the identified problem. If themes are not evident, then
you need to decide carefully whether to continue with the EBNP process or stop
at this point and consider further investigation and research first. It might be that
there is not enough evidence to support a practice change. Rather, the evidence
or lack thereof is supporting the need for more research first.

In the current example, the most significant theme was the need to establish a uniform comprehensive protocol to prevent surgical site infections.
Based on a synthesis of all of the above evidence, critical components of this
protocol include:

- Proper antibiotic choice and administration
- Surgical scrub using nonalcohol-based 2% CHG
- Use of clipping for any hair removal
- Maintaining normothermia through warming
- Targeting early return to normoglycemia by establishing insulin
  protocol
- Proper scrub technique
- Continuing education and communication with healthcare providers, pa-
  tients, and families
- Monitoring outcomes such as compliance with established protocol and
  surgical site infection rates

Integrating the Evidence with Clinical Expertise and Client Preferences and Values

The next level of evidence to be synthesized and added is clinical expertise
and patient preferences and values. Strategies to incorporate clinical expertise and patient values and needs have already been discussed with the earlier
example in this chapter. To tailor this protocol to an individual organization,

it is important to find out if any current protocols exist and the history of such protocols. As with the other example, to ensure a thorough analysis of clinical expertise available, a multidisciplinary approach should be used. For the current issue of surgical site infection, experts might include representation from staff nurses who work in the preoperative and postoperative areas, surgeons, anesthesiologists, pharmacists, administration, infection control, and a recent family member and/or patient. In this particular case, a meeting could be held to ask everyone for his or her input and expert opinion regarding the issue. To incorporate patient needs and preferences, individual or group interviews could be done with past surgical patients and their families. This could be done at discharge or at the first postoperative visit at the provider's office in the form of a short survey or quick semistructured interview. To facilitate synthesis and identification of themes across these interviews, the same slate of questions should be used. Sample interview questions are presented in Table 9-1. Lastly, look to see if the literature includes ideas of how to incorporate patient preferences and needs. For example, Burnett et al. (2009) found that patients were poorly communicated with verbally and never received any written communication. Burnett et al. stress the need to involve patients in the design and evaluation of systems change and information that will improve patient experience. They also stress the need to incorporate patient views appropriately within the organization. To do this Blum (2009) recommends the use of huddle rounds where the care team meets with the patient and their family to discuss plan of care, progress, test results, and changes in condition.

Developing the Proposed Practice Change in Detail

As with the first example presented in this chapter, representation by the target population from the inception of the problem/issue is critical for buy-in and active participation. These individuals can serve as champions during the implementation of the practice change.

Just like the earlier example, this step is the point where decisions are made about who will receive the practice change, what it will entail, when it will happen, where it will take place, and how it will take place.

Who Will Receive the Practice Change?

The target population of the practice change is the preoperative, surgery, recovery, and intensive care nurses, anesthesiologists, surgeons, pharmacists, and infection control staff.

What Is the Practice Change?

Based on input from clinical experts, development of a safety team consisting of representatives from the above categories will provide oversight for the implementation of the practice change. This team may consist of all if not at least part of the original evidence-based nursing practice committee. This team's primary goal will be to propose policy that incorporates the use of the newly developed checklist, provide in-service education to all involved professionals and staff, and to facilitate implementation and evaluation of outcomes. Critical components of this checklist along with examples (not a comprehensive inclusion of all evidence) of supporting evidence include:

- Proper antibiotic choice
  - Choosing the appropriate prophylactic antibiotic prior to surgery is imperative to decrease the incidence of surgical site infections. Haycock et al. (2005) provides one of the sources of evidence for this intervention (Lyons et al. 2009). Haycock et al. describes the recommended choice of antibiotics for patients prior to cardiac surgery as cefazolin 1 g. For those patients with a history of penicillin allergy, the recommended antibiotic is vancomycin. Lyons, et al. also provides an excerpt from a pocket guide used by surgeons at Johns Hopkins Hospital. This pocket guide provides the recommended preoperative antibiotics for a particular surgery. Compliance with this measure will be conducted by a chart audit to see if the correct antibiotic was given.
- Proper antibiotic administration
  - A large percentage of surgical site infections are preventable with appropriate use of prophylactic antibiotics. The antibiotic should be given prior to the initial incision to ensure adequate concentration. Peterson (2002) shares that the American Society of Health-System Pharmacists' guidelines recommend administration between 30 minutes and 1 hour prior to surgery. The CDC recommends 1-hour preincision to be the most effective (Hobson, 2009). Compliance with this measure will be done by a chart audit to see if antibiotic was given at the appropriate time.
  - Redosing based on CDC guidelines is necessary to maintain therapeutic levels of the agent throughout the operation and will be based on initial administration 1 hour preincision (Hobson, 2009). The circulating nurse will report the redosing schedule to the PACU nurse who will report the schedule to the inpatient unit nurse (intensive care or medical-surgical). This schedule will be verified with the pharmacy to ensure consistency and accuracy of administration (Lyons et al., 2009). Compliance with this measure would be conducted by a chart audit to see if correct redosing of the antibiotic had occurred.
  - For most procedures, prophylactic antibiotics will be discontinued within 24 hours of the surgery end time. For cardiac surgeries, this time will be extended to 48 hours based on input and evidence supported by

groups such as the Society of Thoracic Surgeons (Daniels, 2007). Evidence found by Lyons et al. (2009) supports the need for a preprinted set of orders and/or protocols to standardize the process. Compliance with this measure will be conducted by a chart audit to see if the antibiotic has been discontinued as per checklist.

- Surgical scrub using nonalcohol based 2% chlorhexidine (CHG)
  - In a study by Eiselt (2009), surgical site infections decreased by 3.19–1.59% after implementation of the 2% CHG cleansing cloth. This solution has been shown to reduce bacterial counts of acinetobacter and methycillin-resistant *Staphylococcus aureus* (MRSA) by 99.9%. The cloth is easy to use, which can lead to better compliance by patients. After implementing the use of 2% CHG in one hospital, the annual savings came to $348,923 (Rhee, 2008). Compliance with this measure will include chart audit of documentation of use of 2% CHG.
- Use of clipping for any hair removal
  - Lyons et al. (2009) shares several studies to support the use of clipping versus shaving. Studies have shown that shaving with a razor creates small nicks in the skin allowing organisms to colonize and lead to infection. Hair removal should be performed no sooner than 2 hours prior to surgery. The CDC recommends, "If hair is removed, remove immediately before the operation, preferably with electric clippers" (Hobson, 2009). The American Journal of Nursing (2006) reports the following on behalf of the Joanna Briggs Institute, "A randomized study of 1980 patients compared shaving with electrical clippers the night before surgery on the outcome of mediastinitis after coronary bypass surgery. The results were statistically significant in favor of clipping ($p = 0.024$)." Compliance with this measure will be through chart audit for documentation of clipping versus shaving.
- Maintaining normothermia through warming
  - Melling et al. (2001) have found in their study that warming a patient 30 minutes preoperatively reduces surgical site infection by 5–14%. In an interview conducted by Lyons (2009) at her facility, it was found that standard practice included keeping a surgical patient's body temperature at 36°C. Methods used to keep patients at this temperature include blankets from warmers, using a Bair Hugger blanket, or placing warm packs on the patient. Compliance with this measure will be through chart audit to check for documentation of body temperature before, during, and after the surgical procedure, including what interventions were used, if any, to promote warming.

- Targeting early return to normoglycemia by establishing insulin protocol
  - Lyons et al. (2009) cite Haycock et al. (2005) once more to support the importance of this intervention. An average of 10 hours was needed for patients to reach target blood glucose in one study of cardiac surgery patients. Revisions were made to the protocol that included an aggressive approach following surgery to reach the target range. With this more aggressive approach, the average time to target range was reduced to 5.2 hours (Haycock et al., 2005). Compliance data will include mean hourly glucose levels, transition to subcutaneous dosing regimen, comorbidities, hours to target range, and any hypoglycemic event.
- Proper scrub technique
  - Lyons et al. (2009) cite Hsieh et al. (2006) as support for this proposed intervention. Hsieh et al. (2006) recommends that the length of time spent on surgical scrubs should last approximately 5 minutes and shares CDC's recommendations to scrub from the elbows down with a scrubbing duration of 2–6 minutes. Compliance with this measure will include periodic observation of surgical staff.
- Continuing education and communication with healthcare providers, patients, and families
  - Evidence shared to support this intervention includes Burnett et al. (2009) and Blum (2009). Burnett et al. (2009) makes an argument for including patients in the design and evaluation of systems change. Blum (2009) advocates for "huddle rounds." Huddle rounds occur once daily, where the care team meets with the patient and their family to discuss the plan of care, progress, test results, and changes in condition. Patients are encouraged to become active participants through asking questions and voicing concerns. Compliance will be measured by patient and staff satisfaction surveys.
- Monitoring outcomes such as compliance with established protocol and surgical site infection rates
  - Compliance with this new protocol/checklist is critical to its success. Specific examples of compliance measures were provided within each checklist intervention previously mentioned.
  - Surgical site infection rates will be measured before implementation of this new practice change and at specific intervals following implementation. The infection control nurse/staff will also serve a critical role by assessing for signs of surgical site infection on a daily basis.

When Will the Intervention Happen?

Implementation of the new surgical site infection checklist will occur through mandatory in-service education conducted by the evidence-based practice/safety team after administrative and/or organizational approval. These in-services will be conducted over a 4-week period on all shifts including weekends. They will be offered a minimum of four times each week. After the initial rollout of the practice change, the education will be formatted into an online self-study module for ease of continuing education and new employee orientation.

Where Will It Happen?

To facilitate accessibility and ease of attendance, the initial education will be done face to face in an onsite classroom/conference room setting.

How Will It Happen?

Since this will be a mandatory face-to-face education, all involved staff will be paid to attend. The safety team will conduct education. A knowledge test will be given before and after to evaluate level of knowledge gained. Refreshments will be provided along with door prizes to encourage attendance.

Feasibility Issues

Feasibility includes such things as costs, time, and needed resources. A budget, timeline, and list of needed resources need to be developed. For the current issue of implementation of the new surgical site infection prevention checklist, the following costs need to be calculated:

Development of the evidence-based/safety team committee:

- Communication costs (mail, phone calls, flyers, posters)
- Salary for any committee members that are staff to attend meetings
- Refreshments for meetings
- Room to have meetings
- Resources to retrieve the needed evidence (librarian, computer data bases, copying costs)

Implementation of the checklist/policy:

- Salaries for staff to attend educational sessions
- Costs of marketing policy change/checklist
- Room to have educational sessions
- Refreshments if any during mandatory educational sessions
- Cost of door prizes
- Pre- and posttest survey regarding knowledge and attitudes over the practice change

Evaluation of the visitation policy:

- Involved staff and patient/family satisfaction surveys
- Salary of personnel tasked to collect, analyze, and report outcome data

Evaluating the Practice Change

Outcome measures must be identified in order to evaluate the effectiveness of any practice change. For this example, a knowledge test will be administered prior to and immediately following the education to evaluate knowledge gained. Surgical site infection rate, collected on a monthly basis, will be evaluated after 3 months. This rate will be compared to the baseline rate. Three months after implementation of the new checklist/policy, a written satisfaction survey will be conducted with both involved staff and patients/families to see how well they like the checklist and how it influenced the quality of care. Based on the results of these outcomes, the checklist/policy will continue as initially implemented or be revised if improvement has not occurred. For the first year, outcomes will be measured every 3 months and action taken if needed. Then, collection of outcomes can occur on a biannual basis.

Marketing the Practice Change and Strategies for Successful Implementation

Marketing and obtaining buy-in for the practice change are crucial to its success. Including representation from all stakeholders from the inception of any practice change idea will facilitate adoption of the change. In this particular evidence-based practice project, stakeholders include nurses taking care of surgical patients, anesthesiologists, infection control staff, surgeons, pharmacists, and potentially interested past patients/consumers. Keeping stakeholders informed throughout the process, asking for feedback, encouraging positive talk among the rest of the staff that will be involved, getting administrative support, and publicizing the positives that the change will cause are all ideas to consider. The most effective mode of communication is word of mouth using champions for the cause. Other strategies include email, posters, flyers, and notice of mandatory education sessions. A well-planned organized rollout of the practice change is important to its success. A thorough investigation, critique, and synthesis of all of the evidence will go a long way in winning over stakeholders.

Sustainability of Practice Change

Continued monitoring and reinforcement of the practice change is important for sustainability. As mentioned, outcomes will be measured monthly for the first 3 months, then every 6 months thereafter. Revision to the checklist based on outcomes and continued follow-up will be proposed. Keeping current on best practices and current research will help inform any revisions that needs to be done.

REFERENCES

American Journal of Nursing. (2006). Preoperative hair removal and surgical site infection: Long accepted practices aren't always best. *American Journal of Nursing, 106,* 64II–64NN.

Berwick, D. M., & Kotagal, M. (2004, August 11). Restricted visiting hours in ICUs: Time to change. *Jornal of the American Medical Association, 292*(6), 736–737.

Blum, K. (2009). Including patients and families in the conversation. *Dome, 60,* 2.

Buonocore, D. (2004). Leadership in action: Creating a change in practice. *AACN Clinical Issues: Advanced Practice in Acute & Critical Care, 15*(2), 170–181.

Burnett, E., Lee, K., Rushmer, R., Ellis, M., Noble, M., & Davey, P. (2009). Healthcare-associated infection and the patient experience: A qualitative study using patient interviews. *Journal of Hospital Infection, 74,* 42–47.

Center for Innovation in Quality Patient Care. (2009). *Fact sheet.* Retrieved from http://www. hopkinsmedicine.org/innovation_quality_patient_care/.

Daniels, S. (2007). Protecting patients from harm: Improving hospital care for surgical patients. *Nursing, 37,* 36–41.

DeBaun, B. (2008). Evaluation of the antimicrobial properties of an alcohol-free 2% chlorhexidine gluconate solution. *Association of Peri-operative Registered Nurses, 87,* 925–933.

Eiselt, D. (2009). Presurgical skin preparation with a novel 2% chlorhexidine gluconate cloth reduces rates of surgical site infection in orthopedic surgical patients. *Orthopedic Nursing, 28,* 141–145.

Gary, J. (2007, June). *Addressing visitation in critical care: An evidence-based nursing practice project.* PowerPoint presentation as part of completion of Nursing 598 Course for the University of Phoenix Online Nursing Program.

Haycock, C., Laser, C., Keuth, J., Montefour, K., Wilson, M., Austin, K., et al. (2005). Implementing evidence-based practice findings to decrease postoperative sterna wound infections following open heart surgery. *Journal of Cardiovascular Nursing, 20,* 299–305.

Hobson, D. (2009). *Six steps to prevent surgical site infection.* Retrieved from http://www. hopkinsmedicine.org/innovation_quality_patient_care/.

Hsieh, H., Chiu, H., & Lee, F. (2006). Surgical hand scrubs in relation to microbial counts: Systematic literature review. *Journal of Advanced Nursing, 55,* 68–78.

The Joint Commission (2009). *Surgical care improvement project core measure set.* Retrieved from http:///www.jointcommission.org/PerformanceMeasurement/PerformanceMeasurement/SCIP+Core+Measure+Set.htm.

Koopman, E., Nix, D., Erstad, B., Demeure, M., Hayes, M., Ruth, J., et al. (2007). End-of-procedure cefazolin concentrations after administration for prevention of surgical-site infection. *American Journal of Health-System Pharmacy, 64,* 1927–1934.

Lee, M. D., Friedenberg, A. S., Mukpo, D. H., Conray, K., Palmisciano, A., & Levy, M. M. (2007). Visiting hours policies in New England intensive care units: Strategies for improvement. *Critical Care Medicine 35*(2), 497–499.

Livesay, S., Gilliam, A., Mokracek, M., Sebastian, S., & Hickey, J. V. (2005). Nurses' perception of open visiting hours in neuroscience intensive care unit. *Journal of Nursing Care Quality, 20*(2), 182–189.

Lyons, H., Hamburg, M., Bolden, T., Arumugam, M., & Book, C. (2009). Preventing surgical site infection: An evidence-based nursing practice project. Completed November, 23, 2009 for the University of Phoenix Online Nursing Program, Nursing 518 Course.

Melling, A., Ali, B., Scott, E., & Leaper, D. (2001). Effects of preoperative warming on the incidence of wound infection after clean surgery: A randomized controlled trial. *Lancet, 358,* 8786–8880.

Peterson, C. (2002). Surgical-grade stainless steel: When to administer antibiotics; medication labels; mixing medications; bioburden. *Association of Peri-operative Registered Nurses Journal, 76,* 1080–1083.

Rhee, H., & Harris, B. (2008). *Reducing surgical site infections.* Retrieved from http://www.infectioncontroltoday.com/articles/reducing-surgical-infections.html.

Roland, P., Russell, J., Richards, K. P., & Sullivan, S. C. (2001, January). Visitation in critical care: Processes and outcomes of a performance improvement initiative. *Journal of Nursing Care Quality, 15*(2), 18–26.

Sims, J., & Miracle, V. (2006). A look at critical care visitation. *Dimensions of Critical Care Nursing, 25,* 175–180.

White, S. K., & Edwards, R. J. (2006, August). Visitation guidelines promote safe, satisfying environments. *Nursing Management. 37*(8), 20–24.

CHAPTER 10

Planned Change in Evidence-Based Nursing Practice

You have completed all of the work in preparation for evidence-based nursing practice (EBNP) change, and you are ready to implement it, but you find that no one is amenable to what you have to offer. Now what? Most textbooks on EBNP stop short in preparing you for the implementation and evaluation steps. However, it is the opinion of this author that these steps are just as critical to the process as any other step. Why bother to do the work if you cannot implement it?

Leeman, Jackson, and Sandelowski (2006) examined how well research reports facilitated the transfer of findings into practice. Content analysis of 46 reports of diabetes self-management interventions published between 1993 and 2004 found that limited information was provided to guide clinicians in applying the proposed interventions in practice. Specifically, limited information was provided to potential users on the target population; expertise and training required to deliver the intervention; the intervention protocol; and the process of adapting and implementing interventions in practice settings (Leeman et al., 2006).

Translation of research and EBNP findings into practice can be very difficult to do and requires knowledge of change theory. Several theories of planned change exist in the literature, but two of the more common and frequently used that are relevant to EBNP implementation are Rogers' Diffusion of Innovations theory (Rogers, 2003) and Lewin's Model of Planned Change (Lewin, 1972). Lewin's principles were discussed in Chapter 9 with the EBNP visitation policy. This chapter will focus on the relationship of Rogers' Diffusion of Innovations theory to EBNP by also using the evidence-based visitation policy change discussed in Chapter 9.

ROGERS' DIFFUSION OF INNOVATIONS THEORY

Rogers' theory has been applied throughout the world with a variety of disciplines. Even though the original primary focus was technology and diffusion of technological innovations, the theory has also been applied to disciplines such as political science, public health, communications, history, economics, technology, education, and more recently, nursing. Within nursing, it has been used particularly with public health and school health. Four main elements in the Diffusion of Innovations theory are innovation, communication channels, time, and social system.

Innovation

Rogers describes an innovation in the following way: "An innovation is an idea, practice, or project that is perceived as new by an individual or other unit of adoption" (Rogers, 2003, p. 12). The newness characteristic of an adoption is related to three of the steps (knowledge, persuasion, and decision) of the innovation–decision process discussed in more detail later. Uncertainty is a significant obstacle to the adoption of innovation. To reduce this uncertainty, involved individuals should be informed about its advantages and disadvantages from the beginning.

Communication Channels

Rogers defines communication as "a process in which participants create and share information with one another in order to reach a mutual understanding" (p. 5). This communication occurs through channels between individuals, groups, or organizations. Diffusion is a specific kind of communication that includes an innovation, a target population (individual, group, organization), and a communication channel (Rogers, 2003). Examples of communication channels are word of mouth, posters, email, etc. He further shares that "diffusion is a very social process that involves interpersonal communication relationships" (p. 19). Communication channels can be categorized as more local or more external. External sources are more important at the knowledge stage, whereas internal sources are more important at the persuasion stage of the innovation–decision process (Rogers, 2003).

Time

The time aspect is ignored in most behavioral research (Rogers, 2003). Inclusion of the time dimension by using rate of adoption as part of the innovation–diffusion process is a strength of this theory.

Social System

Rogers defines the social system as a "set of interrelated units engaged in joint problem solving to accomplish a common goal" (p. 23). Structure is "the patterned arrangements of the units of a system" (p. 24). Rogers claims that the nature of the social system affects the individual, group, and/or organization's willingness to adopt the innovation. This is his main criterion for categorizing adopters.

The Innovation–Decision Process

An Uncertainty Reduction Process

Rogers (2003) describes the innovation–decision process as an "uncertainty reduction process." Characteristics or attributes that help decrease this uncertainty include relative advantage, compatibility, complexity, trialability, and observability. The individual, group, or organization's perception of these characteristics predicts the rate of adoption of the innovation.

Relative advantage is the degree to which an innovation is perceived as better than the current practice or idea. Incentives for adoption will support and motivate the individual, group or organization to adopt the innovation. Compatibility is another motivation factor. Compatibility is the degree that the innovation is perceived as consistent with existing values, past experiences, and needs of potential adopters. If the innovation is compatible, then uncertainty decreases, and the rate of adoption increases. Complexity is defined as the degree to which an innovation is perceived as difficult to use. As the level of perceived complexity increases, the level of adoption decreases. Trialability is the degree to which an innovation may be experimented with on a limited basis and is positively related to level of adoption. The trial may lead to reinvention or modification of the innovation. Observability is the degree to which the results of an innovation are visible to others. Role modeling, time for practice and training, and peer observation are positively correlated with innovation adoption. In summary, innovations that offer more relative advantage, compatibility, simplicity, trialability, and observability increase the chances of innovation adoption.

Stages of the Process

This process involves five stages: knowledge, persuasion, decision, implementation, and confirmation. Each stage usually occurs in a sequential fashion. See **Table 10-1** for an overview of the stages of the innovation–decision process and factors that can affect adoption throughout the process.

Knowledge stage In the knowledge stage, an individual, group, or organization learns about the existence of the innovation and seeks information about it. The who, what, when, where, and how questions are asked during this stage. These questions contribute to three forms of knowledge: awareness knowledge, how-to knowledge, and principles knowledge. Awareness knowledge is

Table 10-1   Stages of the Innovation–Decision Process and Influencing Factors

Stages	Factors influencing adoption
Knowledge	Prior conditions: previous practice, norms, felt problems
	Characteristics of the social system: socioeconomic characteristics, communication, personality variables
Persuasion	Perceived characteristics of the innovation: relative advantage, compatibility, complexity, trialability, observability
	Opinions and beliefs by self and opinion leaders
Decision	Ability to try out the innovation (pilot programs)
Implementation	Possible reinvention or modification
Confirmation	Level of support for decision to adopt or not

the knowledge that the innovation exists. It can motivate an individual to want to know more about the innovation. The how-to knowledge is essential for the innovation to be adopted. Principles knowledge is describing how and why an innovation works.

Persuasion stage The persuasion stage occurs when the individual, group, or organization develops a negative or positive attitude toward the innovation. However, this does not always lead to the adoption or rejection of the innovation. While knowledge is cognition (knowing) centered, the persuasion stage is more affect (feeling) centered. Social reinforcement from colleagues, peers, and coworkers affects the individual's opinions and beliefs about the innovation.

Decision stage At the decision stage, the individual, group, or organization chooses to adopt or reject the innovation. If an innovation has a partial trial basis, it is usually adopted more quickly, since this allows a trial run of the innovation within the individual setting to see if it works or not. Rejection can occur at any stage of the innovation–decision process. It can be rejected before trying it out or it can be rejected later after initial acceptance.

Implementation stage At the implementation stage, an innovation is put into practice. Uncertainty about the effectiveness of the outcomes can still be a problem at this stage. This is one point where change agents can be critical to reduce the degree of uncertainty about the outcomes and move the innovation forward. Rogers (2003) defines *reinvention*, which usually happens at this stage, as "the degree to which an innovation is changed or modified by a user in the process of its adoption and implementation" (p. 180). Common facilitators of change identified by Achterberg, Schoonhoven, and Grol (2008) include fit with current practice and possibilities for adjusting the innovation to the user's (adopter's) needs and insights.

Confirmation stage At the confirmation stage, the individual, group, or organization looks for support for the decision to adopt or not. Attitudes are crucial at this stage as they attempt to seek supportive messages that confirm their decision to adopt or not. Depending on the support for their decision, later adoption or discontinuance happens during this stage. Discontinuance may occur because a better innovation was found, or due to lack of effectiveness of the innovation.

Adopter Categories

Rogers (2003) defined the adopter categories as "the classification of members of a social system on the basis of innovativeness" (p. 22). This classification includes innovators, early adopters, early majority, late majority, and laggards.

Innovators Innovators are willing to experience new ideas. They are prepared to cope with unsuccessful innovations and tolerate a certain level of uncertainty of success of the innovation. They are also the ones who usually bring in the innovation from the outside.

Early adopters Early adopters are more likely to hold leadership roles within the social system. These leaders can play a central role at virtually every stage of the innovation process, particularly in keeping the momentum for innovation adoption going forward. Early adopters' attitudes about the innovation are very important since these initial attitudes and evaluations reach others who have not made their decision yet.

Early majority The early majority are viewed as having good interaction with other members of the social system but typically do not serve in leadership roles. Their interpersonal skills and networks are still important in the innovation–diffusion process. They tend to be deliberate in their decision to adopt an innovation and therefore usually take more time than innovators and early adopters.

Late majority The late majority are the ones that typically are skeptical about the innovation and its proposed outcomes. To reduce the uncertainty of the innovation, interpersonal networks of close peers should persuade the late majority to adopt and help them feel that it is safe to adopt.

Laggards As Rogers (2003) shares, laggards prefer the traditional view, and they are more skeptical about innovations and change agents than the late majority. They do not have leadership roles, and their interpersonal networks mainly consist of other members of the same social system. Due to lack of awareness knowledge of the innovations, they first want to make sure that an innovation will work before they adopt it. Therefore, laggards tend to watch and wait to see how successful the innovation is before they adopt. Because of this, laggards' innovation–decision period is relatively long.

ROGERS' DIFFUSION OF INNOVATIONS APPLIED TO EVIDENCE-BASED NURSING PRACTICE

To apply this theory in practice, let us take the first problem identified in Chapter 9 by Gary (2007) and go through the innovation–decision process, bringing some clarity to how this theory can apply to nursing practice issues. Gary (2007) identified dissatisfaction with the current visitation policy in critical care by family members as the problem. Prior conditions as identified by Rogers (2003) include previous practice, felt needs/problems, innovativeness, and norms of the social system. In this example, the current visitation policy was not working, and family members of critical care patients were voicing their concerns. Current policy allows only immediate family to visit four times a day (two 30-minute and two 1-hour visitation sessions) and limits to only four visitors at the bedside at a time. Nurses were currently following the policy, but it was not working for the families. After a thorough investigation, the problem was identified as "restrictive visitation policy for critical care families related to current policy only allowing immediate family to visit four times a day as evidenced by family and patient complaints."

Knowledge Stage

In the knowledge stage, the focus is on details about the problem/issue and what practice change/innovation is available to implement. This step is the point where decisions are made about who will receive the practice change, what it will entail, when it will happen, where it will take place, and how it will take place. In the current example, the "who" would be everyone impacted by a new critical care visitation policy. This may include critical care staff nurses, physicians, administration, patients, family members, clergy, and safety officers to name just a few. The "what" would be the development of an effective visitation policy that all could agree on and support. Ideally, representatives from these areas would have served on a committee early on in the practice change inception. Evidence collection, analysis, and synthesis may have been started by one nurse but for an organizational change to occur would need to be extended to all parties with a vested interest (stakeholders) to achieve buy-in. Awareness knowledge and principles knowledge are acquired initially through collecting and analyzing all forms of evidence including empirical and nonempirical evidence, clinical expertise, and patient preferences. Then, these knowledge types become important again during initial introduction and training of potential adopters that is done through educational sessions in this example.

Persuasion Stage

To facilitate the development of a positive attitude toward the innovation, members of the potential adopters group should be included throughout all phases of the innovation or evidence-based nursing practice change. These individuals can serve as champions for implementation and ultimate success of your project. Using email messages, flyers, and posters to publicize the upcoming implementation of innovation will help prepare and set the stage for adoption. Recruiting peers and respected coworkers to present a positive image and attitude towards the proposed innovation will be a challenge to accomplish but an effective way to promote adoption.

Decision Stage

The decision stage is where the decision is made to adopt or reject the innovation. To obtain buy-in from the rest of involved staff, an educational session can be offered. However, this should not be the first communication with those impacted by such a practice change. Initial communication and requesting ideas related to the problem/issue can be done by focus groups or a written survey. Newsletters, emails, and bulletin boards are methods that can be used to keep staff informed throughout the process along with encouraging ideas and feedback that can be taken back to the visitation policy committee for review and consideration.

Implementation Stage

At the implementation stage, an innovation is placed into practice. Because of its newness, the innovation brings with it some degree of uncertainty as it is diffused. One helpful strategy during this stage is to pilot the innovation to determine its effectiveness and to show potential adopters how it can work. During this time it may be found that the innovation as it was originally created is not working during implementation and needs modification. Rogers

(2003) called this *reinvention* and states that it is very common for this to happen. Reinvention is viewed as a positive thing since it means that there is more of a vested interest in the innovation, and the adopters and potential adopters are becoming more actively involved in its implementation. In this scenario, adopters and potential adopters include not only the staff and providers but also the family and patient. As suggested in Chapter 9, involving the family and patient if possible is important to assess their needs and preferences and give them an opportunity to reinvent the innovation. A representative family member can join other involved parties for a focus group discussion regarding the innovation and what modifications if any need to be made. Interviews with family members and patients are another strategy discussed in Chapter 9.

Confirmation Stage

During the confirmation stage, the individual, group, or organization looks for support for their decision. This could include a written satisfaction survey conducted with both nurses and patients/families to see how well they liked the visitation policy. Further, focus groups with staff/nurses and a sample of individual patient/family interviews can be done. Based on the results of these outcomes, the visitation policy will continue as implemented, be reinvented as needed, or be discontinued and replaced with another one. Depending on the innovation, it can even be rejected totally.

Factors Impacting Rate of Adoption of Evidence-Based Practice Change

Attributes of Innovations

As discussed earlier in this chapter, Rogers proposes five attributes or characteristics of innovations that help to decrease the uncertainty about an innovation: relative advantage, compatibility, complexity, trialability, and observability. The strongest predictor of the rate of adoption of an innovation is relative advantage.

Relative advantage To influence relative advantage in this visitation policy scenario, the value of a liberal visitation policy needs to be communicated strongly to the potential adopters. Advantages such as more satisfied patients and families, less time spent on complaints, and increased opportunity to educate and communicate with family members can be emphasized. From an organizational perspective, the organization can pride itself on adopting the best practice based on available evidence. Other incentives can include awards, monetary payment, and recognition to increase motivation for innovation adoption.

Compatibility Even though compatibility is similar to relative advantage, there are some conceptual differences. The innovation needs to be compatible with the potential adopters' values and beliefs. With the visitation policy scenario, if staff, providers, administration, etc. do not see the value in this change or disagree with it, it will affect the rate of diffusion. For example, the nurse who disagrees with the innovation may try to get others to disagree with it by speaking negatively about it. They may even refuse to follow the policy change. On the other hand, if the policy change is compatible with the nurse's values, they will most likely advocate for its implementation and become a champion of the cause. Again, as already discussed, it is critical that these champions be viewed as credible and respected by the potential adopters.

Complexity The more complex the innovation is perceived to be, the less readily the innovation will be adopted. As proposed in the EBNP scenario, educational sessions will take place to discuss how the new policy will be adopted and how that policy will translate into everyday practice. An argument could be made that the new policy/innovation is less difficult than the current one because adopters will have to do less policing to enforce the more rigid original visitation policy.

Trialability Allowing the staff to pilot the new visitation would be trialability in Rogers' (2003) language. The more an innovation is tried, the faster its final adoption. Reinvention, as discussed earlier with implementation, is a possibility because of these trials. For example, the new visitation policy could be implemented on just one shift for a period of 2 months and then reevaluated.

Observability As discussed by Rogers (2003), observability is the degree to which the results of an innovation are visible to others. This can be done through role modeling of the policy implementation by early adopters so that other potential adopters see how it can be implemented successfully. This will promote eventual adoption of the new visitation policy.

Categories of Adopters

Rogers (2003, p. 22) defined the adopter categories as "the classification of members of a social system on the basis of innovativeness." Innovativeness is the degree of adoption relative to others within the target system. Categories of adopters include innovators, early adopters, early majority, late majority, and laggards. Based on his work, the majority of adopters fall within the early majority and late majority categories.

Innovators Innovators are open to experience new ideas and can cope with a level of uncertainty about the innovation at the beginning. They are usually the ones who bring the new idea to the table, oftentimes from outside the system. In the visitation policy example, the primary innovator was a graduate nursing student who holds an administrative position within the system. The idea came partially from a course requirement to develop an evidence-based nursing practice change project. Therefore, the innovation was started from outside of the system. Support from the evidence gleaned from both outside and inside the system also contributed to the innovation idea.

Early adopters Early adopters are likely to hold leadership roles within the system and thus can play a critical role at every stage of the innovation–decision process. Leadership drives the vision and allocates the support through both human and material resources. Without true adoption and commitment of nurse leaders, the program will lack resilience and credibility (Newhouse, 2006). Thus, early attitudes about the innovation by these role models are important. These role models act as opinion leaders within their social system and can be important determinants of a rapid rate of diffusion and sustained behavioral change (Valente & Davis, 1999). If the early adopters approve the innovation, this will lead to an increase in adoption rate by others. So, by communicating their support and expectation that others will use the new visitation policy, they assist with the adoption process.

Early majority Typically, the early majority does not have leadership roles within the system, but they do have good communication skills and interactions with others. Diffusion of the innovation into this group is critical to get adoption by the overall majority involved. In a normal distribution of the adopter categories, Rogers (2003) includes 34% of the potential adopters as the early majority. Champions, identified by the early adopters within this early majority, are critical to an innovation's success. Thus, staff and possibly family members within the critical care unit can be identified as champions for the cause. Their communication skills and positive working relationships can be utilized to facilitate adoption by the rest of group. Informal meetings between them and small groups of staff would be a strategy with potential success.

Late majority As with the early majority, the late majority include approximately 34% of the rest of the potential adopters. They tend to be skeptical of the new innovation and may only adopt because of outside pressure. Again, the interpersonal skills of the early majority can be used to reduce the skepticism and uncertainty of this group. One-on-one discussion between the early majority and late majority to promote the innovation might be a helpful strategy at this point.

Laggards Laggards are even more skeptical than the late majority regarding the innovation. In the visitation policy example, laggards may not become adopters until success of the innovation is proven through the trial or pilot periods of the policy. They may still choose to reject the policy and refuse to implement it. However, other motivating factors (e.g., organizational pressure, family and patient demands, peer pressure) may increase the laggards' perceived relative advantage to adopt the policy change.

Four Main Elements in the Diffusion of Innovation Model

Innovation

The innovation is a new liberal visitation policy for families of critical care patients. Explanation of the what, why, and how are critical to the innovation's success and have been carefully addressed in Chapter 9. Content of the educational sessions also included the potential benefits and problems with the implementation of the new policy.

Communication Channels

As can be seen throughout this chapter, effective communication is paramount for any successful implementation of the new visitation policy. Communication channels from outside sources to inside sources and then from leaders to innovative staff down to the most skeptical is important for diffusion and complete adoption of the new policy. External demands and pressure from administration, peers, patients, and families can also affect the adoption process.

Time

The innovation–decision process, rate of adoption characteristics, and adopter categories all include a time component. The stages of the innovation–decision process follow each other in a time-ordered sequential manner from knowledge to persuasion to decision to implementation to confirmation. Adoption rate relates to the time it takes an individual to adopt an innovation. Characteristics (relative advantage, compatibility, complexity, trialability, observability) of innovations influence this rate of adoption. Categories of adoption (innovators, early adopters, early majority, late majority, laggards) also relate to the time of adoption based on the individual's innovativeness. Time for implementation and adoption of the visitation policy was integrated within the evidence-based nursing practice change in Chapter 9.

Social System

The social system involved in the visitation policy included the hospital, the critical care unit, involved physicians and staff, administrative staff, and critical care patients and families. All key players were included from the inception to the implementation and evaluation of the innovation.

An Example of a Failed Attempt to Diffuse an Innovation

Rogers (2003) provides an excellent example to illustrate the common difficulties when trying to diffuse an innovation throughout a social system. The social system in this case was a Peruvian village, and the innovation was water boiling to prevent the spread of infectious disease among its members. This innovation was identified as a need by the public health service in Peru. However, it would require a major change in thinking for the villagers, who do not understand the relationship of sanitation to illness. A 2-year boiling campaign in a village of 200 families persuaded only 11 housewives to boil water. Rogers shares that the innovation failed because the villagers perceived the innovation as culturally inappropriate. Local tradition links hot foods and liquids with illness. So, why boil water if one is not sick? An important factor for adoption rate of an innovation is its compatibility with the values and beliefs of individuals within the social system. The public health service did not consider this during their diffusion effort. Therefore, it ultimately failed.

Rogers (2003) offers several suggestions for this case that would have prevented failure. First, the public health service worker focused on the wrong housewives to start a diffusion of the practice of boiling water. She focused her attention on a housewife viewed as sickly and a housewife viewed as a social outsider as perceived by the villagers. She ignored the village opinion leaders who could have pushed the rate of adoption significantly. The public health service worker was viewed as an outsider and not deemed credible or trusted by the villagers. Again, identifying the opinion leaders within the village and working through them would have prevented this problem. The public health service worker could not see the situation from the villagers' perspective and did not understand why they were not interested in learning about germ theory. As one of the housewives so profoundly put it, "If germs are so small that they cannot be seen or felt, how can they hurt a grown person?" (Rogers, 2003)

I hope that we as nurses can learn from such a classic example of what not to do. The goal of this book is to provide you with the tools needed to provide evidence-based nursing practice in a way that is practical and understandable. What do you have to lose with so much more to gain? Do you not owe it to your clients to provide the best quality care possible? Why not get started now?

REFERENCES

Achterberg, T., Schoonhoven, L., & Grol, R. (2008). Nursing implementation science: How evidence-based nursing requires evidence-based implementation. *Journal of Nursing Scholarship, 40,* 302–310.

Leeman, J., Jackson, B., & Sandelowski, M. (2006). An evaluation of how well research reports facilitate the use of findings in practice. *Journal of Nursing Scholarship, 38,* 171–177.

Lewin, K. (1972). Quasi-stationary social equilibrium and the problems of permanent change. In N. Margulies & A. P. Raia (Eds.), *Organizational development: Values, process, and technology.* New York, NY: McGraw-Hill.

Newhouse, R. (2006). Creating infrastructure supportive of evidence-based nursing practice: Leadership strategies. *Worldviews on Evidence-Based Nursing, 4,* 21–29.

Rogers, E. (2003). *Diffusion of innovations.* New York, NY: Free Press.

Valente, T., & Davis, R. (1999). Accelerating the diffusion of innovations using opinion leaders. *The Annals of the American Academy of Political and Social Science, 566,* 55–67.

Index

Note: page numbers followed by f or t denote figures or tables respectively.

A

Abstract, analysis of, 84
Academic Center for Evidence-Based Practice (ACE) Star Model, 78–79, 78f
Adopters, categories of, 255–256, 259–261
American Nurses Association Research and Studies Commission, 208
Analysis of variance (ANOVA), 63
Animal research safety principle, 215
Anonymity, human research subject's right to, 214
Applicability factor in qualitative research, 48
Appropriateness criterion for evidence, 224
Attrition in sample during study (dropout rate), 26, 43t
Average deviation (variance) measure of variability, 61–63
Awareness knowledge, 253–254

B

Basic social processes, discovering, 47
Bedside (clinical) nurses, 5, 9, 79, 80
Bell curve (symmetrical) distribution, 56, 56f
Belmont Report, 208, 216

Beneficence principle, 208, 209, 210
Black fathers and support for partners in labor study, 37t, 46
Body mass index and health promotion study, 40
Bracketing to avoid researcher enmeshment, 48t, 49

C

Case study methodology, 38, 46
Categorical measurement scales (nominal and ordinal), 57, 58, 59, 60, 66, 68f
Causality relationships and research design, 39, 40, 43–44
CDSR (Cochrane Database of Systematic Reviews), 12t
Central tendency, measures of, 59–60, 61–62
Champions for marketing practice change, 81, 86, 91, 233, 247, 260
Change theory, 80, 91, 252–262
Children and human research subjects' rights, 209
Chi-square (χ^2) test, 65
CINAHL (cumulative index of the nursing and allied health) database, 8, 19, 84
Clinical expertise as EBNP resource, 6, 86, 87t, 223–224, 232–233, 234t
Clinical (bedside) nurses, 5, 9, 79, 80

Clinical practice, applying EBNP to. *See* Implementing EBNP
Clinical vs statistical significance, 72
Cochrane, Archie, 223
Cochrane Collaboration, 223
Cochrane Database of Systematic Reviews (CDSR), 12t
Cochrane Library, 12t
Communication channels, importance for change process, 252, 261
Comparative descriptive research design, 39
Compatibility in innovation adoption, 253, 259
Competency of investigator, principle of, 214–215
Complex vs simple hypotheses, 22
Complexity in innovation adoption, 253, 259
Concept, defined, 20
Conduct and Use of Research in Nursing (CURN), 4, 5
Confidentiality, human research subject's right to, 214
Confirmation stage of innovation adoption, 255, 258
Confounding/extraneous variables, 23–24
Consistency in qualitative research, 50
Constant comparative method, 47, 109
Construct, defined, 20
Construct validity, 28–29
Content analysis, 86–87, 232
Content validity, 28–29
Content validity index (CVI), 29
Continuous (interval and ratio) measurement scales, 57, 58, 66, 69–70f
Continuous vs dichotomous variables, 21
Controlling for confounding variables, 24
Convenience sampling, 25
Convergent validity, 29
Cookbook approach to patient care, avoiding, 224–225
Core variables, identifying, 47
Correlation coefficient, 63, 64f, 65
Correlational study, 38, 39–40, 67t
Cost-effectiveness factor, 226

Costs/resources for practice change, assessing, 4, 88–89, 89f, 224, 235
Covariance, 24
Cronbach's alpha, 29
Cultural competence, 210
CURN (Conduct and Use of Research in Nursing), 4, 5
CVI (content validity index), 29

D

DARE (Database of Abstracts of Reviews of Effectiveness), 12t
Data analysis
    choosing statistical tests, 66–71, 68–70f
    descriptive statistics, 54, 55–62
    inferential statistics, 54, 62–66
    interpreting statistical tests, 71–72
    introduction, 53–54
    overview, 4
    qualitative research, 4, 109, 111
    quantitative research, 4, 30–31, 53–71, 100, 103–104
Data collection
    overview, 3–4
    qualitative research, 108, 111
    quantitative research, 27–30, 100, 103
    and study instruments, 28–30, 43t, 50
Data saturation, 49–50
Database of Abstracts of Reviews of Effectiveness (DARE), 12t
Databases, 8, 12t, 18–19, 84
Decision stage of innovation adoption, 254, 257
Declaration of Helsinki, 208
Dependent vs independent variables, 21–22, 30–31
Descriptive research design, 21, 38–39, 67t, 193
Descriptive statistics, 54, 55–62
Design, research project, 3, 35–43. *See also* Qualitative research; Quantitative research
Dichotomous vs continuous variables, 21
Diffusion of Innovations theory, 91, 252–262
Directional vs nondirectional hypotheses, 22

Discriminant validity, 29
Dissemination of findings, 4, 32
Distribution, statistical, 55–56, 56–57f, 60, 62, 65
Distribution-free statistical tests, 65–66
Divergent validity, 29
"Doing no harm" ethical principle, 209, 210

E
Early adopters, 255, 260
Early majority, 255, 260
EBM (evidence-based medicine), 5–6
EBNP (evidence-based nursing practice).
    See also Implementing EBNP
    ethical considerations, 222–226
    introduction, 5–6
    models for, 75–82
    myths about, 7–10
    vs nursing research, 7, 7t
    overcoming barriers to using, 10–14
    surgical site infection process example, 237–248
    10-step process, 81, 82t
    variety of resources for, 11, 12t
    visitation policy dissatisfaction in patients and families example, 229–237
EBP (evidence-based practice), 5–6
Effect size, analyzing, 27
Effectiveness criterion for evidence, 224
Elite bias, 50
Emergent design, 45, 46, 110
Empirical research study analysis.
    See also Qualitative research;
    Quantitative research
    as EBNP resource, 6
    overview, 83–85, 95, 96–97t
    qualitative sample articles, 104–112, 141–164, 171–183
    quantitative sample articles, 98–104, 113–121, 123–138
    steps and points division, 96–97t, 105–106t
    visitation policy example, 230
Ethics in research
    EBNP vs research and, 222–223
    ethical violations case study, 215–216

ethics defined, 207
    guidelines for nurses, 208–215
    historical perspective, 207–208
    informed consent, 25, 207, 209, 210t, 211–213t
    IRB's role, 208, 216–219, 220–221t
    potential pitfalls for EBNP, 223–226
    present-day challenges, 219, 222
    rights of human subjects, 207–214
    and volunteer nature of sample, 26
Ethnography, 47
Evaluation
    importance of research study, 10
    of practice change, 90, 236, 247
Evidence and EBNP, 7–8, 223
Evidence-based medicine (EBM), 5–6
Evidence-based nursing practice (EBNP).
    See EBNP (evidence-based nursing practice)
Evidence-based practice (EBP), 5–6
Evidence-Based Practice Model for Staff Nurses, 80
Exemplar cases, 46, 48t
Exempt review, 217, 218–219t
Exercise motivation for Mexican-American adults study, 50–51
Expedited review, 217, 220–221t
Experimental research
    confounding variables challenge, 23–24
    deciding on design, 38, 41–42
    elements of, 21
    vs nonexperimental quantitative design, 66–67t
    quantitative research analysis examples, 102
    vs quasi-experimental, 40
    randomized controlled trials (RCTs), 31, 41, 223
    results interpretation, 71–72
    sampling methods, 33
Expert panel, 50
External validity, 42–44, 49
Extraneous/confounding variables, 23–24

F
Factor-isolating research questions, 38–39
Factor-relating research questions, 39–40

Fair treatment, human research subject's
    right to, 213–214
Fatigue and sleep quality in nurses study
    example, 193–197
Feasibility issues, 4, 88–90, 224, 235
Fieldwork phase of ethnographic
    research, 47
Findings/recommendations
    determining, 4
    dissemination of, 4, 32
    generalizability of, 42–44, 49
    quantitative research process, 31
Focused ethnography, 110
Frequency distributions, 55–56
Full board review, 219

G
Gantt chart, 89–90, 90f
Generalizability of research findings,
    42–44, 49
"Going native" problem in qualitative
    research, 50
Grounded theory, 20, 47, 107

H
Hand washing compliance study
    (Creedon), 3, 8, 20, 21, 28, 30
Hand-hygiene intervention study (Siegel &
    Korniewicz), 40–41
Hawthorn effect, 92
Health Insurance Portability and
    Accountability Act (HIPAA), 208
Heller, Jean, 215
Heparin, 8
Heterogeneous vs homogeneous samples,
    26
HIPAA (Health Insurance Portability and
    Accountability Act), 208
Histogram, 55f
History threat to internal validity, 43t
Holistic fallacy, 50
Homogeneous vs heterogeneous samples, 26
Hope in women with advanced ovarian
    cancer study, 47
How-to knowledge, 254
Human as instrument in qualitative
    research, 44

Human subject research, ethical
    considerations. See Ethics in research
Hypotheses. See Research questions/
    hypotheses

I
Identification of practice problem/issue, 2,
    83, 229–230, 237–238
Implementation stage of innovation
    adoption, 255, 257–258
Implementing EBNP
    EBNP models, 75–82
    empirical research analysis, 85
    evaluation of practice change, 90, 236,
        247
    evidence appraisal, 83–85, 230–232,
        238–241
    feasibility issues, 88–90, 246–247
    identifying clinical practice problem, 83,
        229–230, 237–238
    integrating evidence with clinical
        situation, 86, 87t, 232–233, 234t,
        241–242
    introduction, 75
    marketing of practice change, 81, 86, 91,
        233, 236, 247, 260
    planned change process, 251–262
    proposed practice change development,
        86, 88, 233, 234–235, 242–246
    strategies for, 91, 236–237
    summarizing across evidence, 85–86,
        232, 241
    sustainability of practice change, 91–92,
        237, 247
    10 steps for creating changes, 82t
Independent vs dependent variables,
    21–22, 30–31
Inferential statistics, 54, 62–66
Informed consent, 25, 207, 209, 210t,
    211–213t
Innovation, defined, 252
Innovation–decision process, 253–259, 254t
Innovators, 255, 259–260
Institutional review boards (IRBs), 208,
    216–219, 220–221t
Instrumentation threat to internal
    validity, 43t

Instruments, study
  data collection, 28–30, 43t, 50
  measurement scales, 56–62, 66, 68–70f
  qualitative research examples, 108,
    111
  quantitative research examples, 99–100,
    103
Integrity of research process, principle
  of, 214
Internal validity, 29, 42, 48, 49
Interval measurement scale, 57, 69–70f
Interview method, 46, 48t
Intuitive, felt knowledge in qualitative
  research, 45, 48t
Iowa model, 76, 77f, 78
IRBs (institutional review boards), 208,
  216–219, 220–221t

J
Joanna Briggs Institute (JBI), 12t, 224
Justice principle, 208

K
Key and Electronic Nursing Journals:
  Characteristics and Database
  Coverage (KENJ), 54
KKI lead paint study, 219
Knowledge stage of innovation adoption,
  253–254, 256–257

L
Laggards, 256, 261
Late majority, 256, 260
Levels of measurement, 56–58
Lewin's Theory of Change, 236–237
Librarian, literature review role of, 19
Likert scale, 57–58
Literature review
  overview, 2
  process of, 83–85
  qualitative research, 107, 110
  quantitative research, 18–19, 98, 102
Logistical regression, 65–66

M
Magnet hospital program, 9
Mann-Whitney U test, 65

MANOVA (multivariate analysis of
  variance), 63
Marketing of practice change
  champions for, 81, 86, 91, 233, 247, 260
  importance of, 236
Matching on confounding variable, 24
Maturation threat to internal validity, 43t
Mean (average) central tendency measure,
  59, 60, 61–62
Meaningfulness criterion for evidence,
  224
Measurement methods, 56–62, 66, 68–70f
Median central tendency measure, 59, 60
Medical information, protection of, 208
MEDLINE database, 19, 84
Member checking in qualitative research,
  45
Misconduct, responsibility to report
  scientific, 214
Mixed methods approach, 50–51
Mode central tendency measure, 59, 59f
Multiple regression, 63, 65
Multivariate analysis of variance
  (MANOVA), 63

N
The National Commission for the
  Protection of Human Subjects of
  Biomedical and Behavioral Research,
  208
National Quality Measures Clearinghouse,
  12t
Natural setting for qualitative research, 44
Naturalistic vs positivist paradigms in
  nursing research, 35, 36t
Negotiated outcomes in qualitative
  research, 45
Neutrality in qualitative research, 50
Nominal measurement scale, 57, 59, 60, 68f
Nonempirical research analysis, 6, 83–85,
  231
Nonmaleficence principle, 209, 210
Nonnormal (skewed) distributions, 56,
  57f, 60, 65
Nonparametric statistical tests, 65–66
Nonprobability vs probability sampling,
  24–25

Normal (symmetrical) distribution, 56, 56f
Nuremberg Code, 207
Nursing research. *See also* EBNP (evidence-based nursing practice)
  vs EBNP, 7, 7t
  introduction, 1–4
  math/statistics fear of, 10–11
  positivist vs naturalistic paradigms, 35, 36t
  vs research utilization, 7, 7t
  rights of human subjects in, 207–214
  value for nursing practice, 7–8

O

Observability in innovation adoption, 253, 259
Office of Research Integrity, 214
Oral hygiene study, 39
Ordinal measurement scale, 57, 60, 68f
Outcome measures, evaluating, 90

P

P value, interpreting, 71
Paired samples T-test, 63
Paradigm cases, 46, 48t
Parametric statistical tests, 62–65
Participant observation, 46, 47–48, 48t
Patency in peripheral intermitted intravenous devices, 8
Patient preferences and values
  impact as evidence in practice change, 223–224
  in implementation of EBNP, 86
  importance for EBNP, 7, 225
  integration with evidence, 232–233
  sample interview questions, 87t, 234t
Pearson's *r*, 65
Peer debriefing, 50
Percentage distribution, 62
Percentile measure, 62
Persuasion stage of innovation adoption, 254, 257
Phenomenology, 46, 189
Physical activity in ethnic midlife women study example, 198–201
Population, study, defined, 3

Positivist vs naturalistic paradigms in nursing research, 35, 36t
Power analysis, 26–27, 49
Power of the study, defined, 26
Practice, nursing. *See also* Implementing EBNP
  evidence's value for, 7–8
  qualitative design's applicability to, 46–48, 48t
PRECEDE health education theory, 20
Predictive studies, 39
Predictive validity, 29
Primary vs secondary sources, 85
Principles knowledge, 254
Privacy, human research subject's right to, 214
Privacy Rule, HIPAA, 208
Probability vs nonprobability sampling, 24–25
Problem statement
  qualitative research, 106–107, 109–110
  quantitative research, 17, 98, 101
Protection from harm, human research subject's right to, 209, 210
Purpose statement. *See* Research questions/hypotheses
Purposive sampling, 25, 45

Q

Qualitative research
  characteristics of, 36t, 44–45
  data analysis, 4, 30, 109, 111
  data collection, 108, 111
  and design decision, 35, 36–37t, 37
  literature review, 107, 110
  and mixed methods approach, 50–51
  and naturalistic paradigm, 35
  and nursing practice, 46–48, 48t
  overview, 3
  problem statement/purpose statement, 106–107, 109–110
  sample articles, 104–112, 141–164, 171–183, 187–192, 198–201
  sampling techniques, 25
  steps and points for analysis, 105–106t
  strengths and limitations assessment, 109, 112

theoretical/conceptual framework, 20, 107, 110
threats to rigor for, 48–50, 48t, 108, 111
value to EBNP, 223
Quality of patient care, 9, 224–225
Quantitative research
characteristics of, 36t
data analysis, 4, 30–31, 53–71, 100, 103–104
data collection, 27–30, 100, 103
in design decision, 24, 35, 36–37t, 37
experimental, 66–67t, 102
findings/recommendations, 31–32
literature review, 18–19, 98, 102
and mixed methods approach, 50–51
overview, 3
and positivist paradigm, 35
problem statement, 17, 98, 101
research questions/hypotheses, 21–22, 22t, 38–42, 41f, 98, 101
sample articles, 98–104, 113–121, 123–138, 193–197, 201–205
sampling, 24–27, 99
steps and points division for analyzing, 96–97t
strengths and limitations assessment, 31–32, 100–101
theoretical/conceptual framework, 19–21, 98, 102
threats to validity, 42–44, 43t, 99, 102
types of, 37–38
variable identification and control, 23–24, 47, 99, 102–103
Quartile chart, 62
Quasi-experimental research, 21, 38, 40, 67t, 71–72

R
Random selection vs random assignment, 23–24
Randomized controlled trials (RCTs), 31, 41, 223
Randomizing the sample, 23–25, 40
Range measure of variability, 60
Rapid response teams, 8–9
Rate of adoption of change, 252, 258–259, 261

Ratio measurement scale, 58, 69–70f
Reading related literature. *See* Literature review
Regression analysis, 65
Reinvention, 255, 258, 259
Relative advantage in innovation adoption, 253, 258
Reliability of data collection instrument, 28, 29–30, 48, 49
Repeated measures crossover study design, 99
Research design, 3, 35–43. *See also* Qualitative research; Quantitative research
Research questions/hypotheses
error types, 27
identifying, 2
levels of, 38–41
in qualitative research, 106–107, 109–110
in quantitative research, 21–22, 22t, 98, 101
and research design choice, 35, 37, 37t, 38–42, 41f
Research utilization, 4–5, 7, 7t
Resources/costs for practice change, assessing, 88–89, 89f, 224, 235
Respect for diversity ethical principle, 210
Respect for persons principle, 208, 216
Results, interpretation of, 71–72
Reversal theory, 20, 102
Rights of human subjects in nursing research, 207–214
Rigor in qualitative research, 48–50, 48t, 108, 111
Roche, Ellen, 219
Rogers' Diffusion of Innovations theory, 91, 252–262
Rosswurm and Larrabee model, 80

S
Sample/sampling
attrition during study, 26, 43t
overview, 3
purposive sampling, 25, 45
qualitative research, 25, 108, 111
quantitative research, 24–27, 33, 99

Sample/sampling (*continued*)
　　randomizing the sample, 23–25, 40
　　size issue, 25–26, 27, 31, 49
Sarah Cole Hirsh Institute, 12t
Scatter plot, 63, 64f, 65
Secondary vs primary sources, 85
Selection threat to internal validity, 43t
Self-determination, human research
　　subject's right to, 209
Significance, statistical vs clinical, 72
Significance level (alpha), 27, 71
Simple random sampling, 24
Simple vs complex hypotheses, 22
Simulation effectiveness in ACLS training
　　study, 42
Situation-producing questions, 21, 41
Situation-relating questions, 21, 40
Skewed (nonnormal) distributions, 56, 57f,
　　60, 65
Social system's role in change process,
　　252–253, 261–262
Sources for evidence analysis, 84–85
Spearman's rho, 65, 66
Spiritual care study, 20
SPSS (Statistical Package Social
　　Sciences), 55
Stability over time for data collection
　　instrument, 29–30
Staff nurses, 5, 9, 79, 80
Standard deviation measure of variability,
　　60–62
Statistical methods and types, 54, 54t,
　　55–71. *See also* Data analysis
Statistical Package Social Sciences
　　(SPSS), 55
Statistical regression threat to internal
　　validity, 43t
Statistical vs. clinical significance, 72
Stetler model, 75–76
Stratified random sampling, 24–25
Strengths and limitations assessment of
　　research, 31–32, 100–101, 109, 112
Subject burden, 26, 31
Summarizing across the evidence, 85–86,
　　232
Surgical site infection EBNP process
　　example, 237–248

Survey research, 38
Sustainability of practice change, 91–92
Symmetrical (normal) distribution, 56,
　　56f

T

Teenage pregnancy study example,
　　187–192
Tentative application in qualitative
　　research, 45
Testing threat to internal validity, 43t
Test-retest reliability, 29–30
Tests, statistical, 62–71
Theoretical frameworks
　　change theory, 80, 91, 252–262
　　Diffusion of Innovations theory, 91,
　　　252–262
　　ethnography, 47–48
　　grounded theory, 20, 47, 107
　　Lewin's Theory of Change, 236–237
　　overview, 2–3
　　phenomenology, 45, 189
　　PRECEDE health education theory, 20
　　qualitative research, 20, 107, 110
　　quantitative research, 19–21, 98, 102
　　reversal theory, 20, 102
Threats to rigor for qualitative research,
　　48–50, 48t, 108, 111
Threats to validity for quantitative
　　research, 42–44, 43t, 99, 102
Time factor in adoption of change, 252,
　　258–259, 261
Timeline for clinical practice change,
　　89–90, 90f
Trialability in innovation adoption, 253,
　　259
Trustworthiness/rigor criteria, 48–50, 48t,
　　108, 111
Truth-value in qualitative research, 49
T-tests, 63
Tuskegee Syphilis Study, 213, 215
Type I error, 27, 42, 71
Type II error, 27, 42, 71

U

Uncertainty reduction process in
　　innovation adoption, 253, 255, 257–259

United States Public Health Service
(USPHS), 215
US Department of Health and Human
Services, 208
USPSTF-AHRQ, 12t

V
Validity in quantitative research, 42–44,
43t, 99, 102
Validity of data collection instrument,
28–29, 30
Variability, measure of, 60–62
Variables
defined, 21–22
dependent vs independent, 21–22, 30–31
identification and control of, 23–24, 47,
99, 102–103

Variance (average deviation) measure of
variability, 61–63
Visitation policy dissatisfaction in
patients and families example,
229–237, 256–262
Visual analog scale (VAS), 57, 58f

W
Walking adherence and depressive
symptoms in African-American
women study example, 201–205
Wan, Nicole, 219
Western Interstate Commission for Higher
Education (WICHE), 4–5
Wilcoxon signed-rank test, 65
Within-subjects design, 63